THE ROLFING® EXPERIENCE

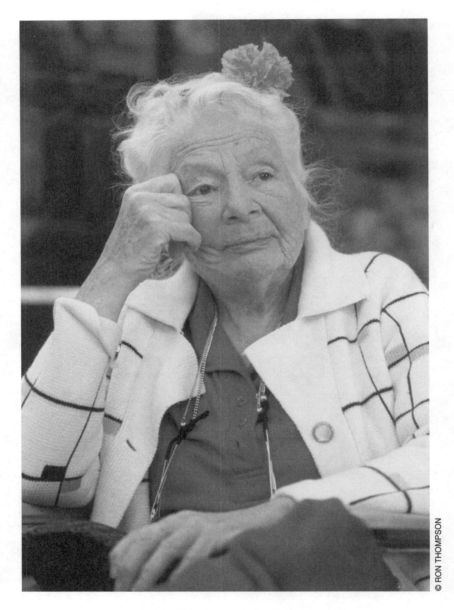

Dr. Ida P. Rolf (1897 – 1979) "The Dreamer."
Photo by Ron Thompson

THE ROLFING® EXPERIENCE

Integration in the Gravity Field

Betsy Sise

HOHM PRESS
Prescott, Arizona

Cover design: Kim Johansen
Layout and design: Tori Bushert

Library of Congress Cataloging in Publication Data:
Sise, Betsy.
   The rolfing experience : integration in the gravity field / Betsy Sise.
        p. cm.
   Includes bibliographical references and index.
   ISBN 1-890772-52-6 (pbk. : alk. paper)
   1. Rolfing. I. Title.
   RC489.R64S57 2005
   615.8'22--dc22

                                        2005020040

HOHM PRESS
P.O. Box 2501
Prescott, AZ 86302
800-381-2700
http://www.hohmpress.com

This book was printed in the U.S.A. on acid-free paper using soy ink.

09 08 07 06 05   5 4 3 2 1

For Peter Melchior my teacher and friend who taught me Rolfing and so much more through his touch, his humor, his wisdom and his presence.

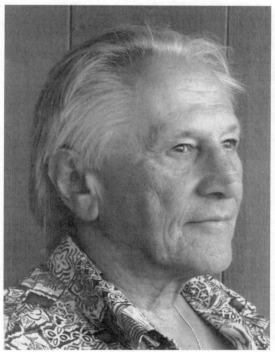

Peter Melchior, 1931 – 2005

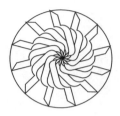

Acknowledgements

To be given my life's work of Rolfing by my first spiritual Teacher, Swami Amar Jyoti, and then to be invited to write a book about it by my present spiritual Teacher, Lee Lozowick, is a piece of synchronicity that defies all expectation. I acknowledge each of them for truly "seeing" me in much the same way Ida Rolf saw people. I am deeply grateful for the tremendous gift of these two Teachers and the Grace with which they appeared in my life. Because of Lee's vision and invitation I had the opportunity to once again meet with each of my four main Rolfing teachers and to walk again the path of my twenty-seven years as a Rolfer in the writing of this book.

My editor Regina Sara Ryan is a writer's gift to publication. Her encouragement and guidance were invaluable. As we worked together I felt a real sense of teamwork, and my trust in her as both editor and friend made the writing of this book that much more enjoyable.

Heartfelt thanks go to all the people who agreed to be interviewed for this book: my four Rolf teachers, Emmett Hutchins, Peter Melchior, Jan Sultan and Tom Wing, as well as Rosemary

Feitis, Jeff Linn, Paul Oertel, Nancy Spanier, Tom Lennon and Sally Sise. Thanks to Jan Sultan for being willing to go a bit out on a limb to express his views, and for the excellent background of knowledge he gave me in my auditing class. Thanks also for our work together on the Admissions Committee and for fun talks in the early days at Tom and Heather Wing's house. Thanks to Tom Wing for seeing me beyond the "dork suit" and for helping me to see at a deeper level by challenging me to take off my glasses when Rolfing. Thanks to Emmett Hutchins for challenging my mind and for all the wonderful opportunities he gave to me through teaching assistantships, trading Rolf sessions, and Rolfing together "four-handed." Thanks also for exuberant times with music and computers at Abbey Place and a grand introduction to Hawaii. Thanks to Peter Melchior for allowing his being to shine so that I often felt met, heart to heart, by just being present with him. From Peter I learned about the elusive "middle layer" of connective tissue and how easily change could happen with the right pressure and awareness. Peter's sense of humor, storytelling and flair for the dramatic made Rolf classes relaxed and enjoyable.

Thanks to Rosemary Feitis for her support through some of the more challenging aspects of writing this book. Her clearheaded view and her close association with Dr. Rolf were especially helpful in collecting background information. Her willingness to read the manuscript and give candid feedback was a real boon.

Thanks to my good friends Paul Oertel and Nancy Spanier for love, support and hospitality when I was in Boulder. Their reading of the manuscript was of special help with particular chapters. I am extremely grateful for their generous sharing of personal experiences in being Rolfed.

Thanks to Tom Lennon for information on alchemy and "the alchemist," and to Jeff Linn for his time and help with some of the historical background of Rolfing and Dr. Rolf.

Thanks to Susan Melchior, Peter's wife, and school director for the Guild for Structural Integration for making the resources of G.S.I. available to me. Her generosity in opening her home to us Rolfers for class parties and gatherings, and for sharing Peter with us were incomparable gifts.

Thanks to Richard Stenstadvold, president of G.S.I., for so graciously and candidly speaking with me of the early days of the Rolf Institute and G.S.I. Special thanks to Richard, Emmett, Wayne Hackett and Howard Carvalho for heartwarming hospitality when I was in Hawaii.

Thanks to the staff of the Rolf Institute and especially to Karna Knapp for loaning me archival videos and making Dr. Rolf's personal library available to me.

Thanks to Kelly and Christina Sell, Rachel Peters, Donna Jo Cross Sutherland, Dan Frazee and Vicki Clay for help with photography. I thank Claire and John Cocke, Alan Goodman and Annie Duggan who also gave assistance with the manuscript. Thanks to Elyse April for the tracing of drawings.

Thanks to my sister Sally Sise, who is also a healing arts practitioner, for a heroine's effort in reading each chapter and giving me feedback as well as much needed encouragement. Thanks to my sister Nancy Auseklis for her support of me and her willingness to be Rolfed. Thanks to my cousin Lelie Sise, a chiropractor, for help with the manuscript. Even though both my parents have passed on I thank my dad, Albert Sise, for instilling in me a sense of adventure, and my mom, Susan Sise, for being behind me no matter what. They would have loved to see their daughter a published author.

Last but not least, thank you to all my clients from whom I have learned so much and to the particular clients who volunteered to write of their experiences being Rolfed.

Disclaimers

The purpose of Rolfing®/Structural Integration (SI) is to balance and align the physical body so that it is supported and maintained by gravity in three-dimensional space. This is done through direct manipulation and education to achieve greater economy and freedom of body movement. Rolfing* is not involved with the treatment of a disease of any kind nor does it substitute for medical diagnosis or treatment when such attention is needed. The Rolfer does not diagnose, prescribe, or treat any illness, disease, or any other physical or mental disorder of a person. Nothing said or done by a Rolfer should be construed as such.

Practitioners of Rolfing/Structural Integration have received extensive training and certification in this work, and the results of this work can be powerful and far reaching. Nothing said in this book should in any way be construed to mean that anyone other than a certified practitioner of Rolfing/SI should attempt to do Rolfing/SI.

The names of clients mentioned in this book have been changed to protect their identity. Many clients' experiences reported are composites of clients with whom the author has worked. The stories quoted at length from interviews were used with the permission of the clients, and one client requested that his own name be used.

* The word "Rolfing" is a service mark of the Rolf Institute of Structural Integration in Boulder, Colorado.

Contents

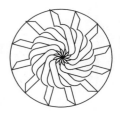

Introduction

This book is about the gift of Rolfing[1] and how it has affected my life and the lives of my clients. I will present Dr. Rolf's ideas and principles as they were given to me from my teachers, giving basic information of how her vision actually works in a body and a being, and how people, myself included, have been affected by her work.

Although Dr. Rolf had a wide circle of students around her in the early days of Rolfing, including Annie Duggan, Ron McComb, Jim Asher, Nicholas French, Joseph Heller, Michael Salveson, Stacey Mills, and Dorothy Nolte, to name a few, I have chosen to focus my interviews for this book with the four principal teachers with whom I trained – Jan Sultan, Tom Wing, Emmett Hutchins and Peter Melchior – each of whom were trained directly by Ida Rolf. Rosemary Feitis, who was Dr. Rolf's secretary for four years, also provided me with a wealth of information on the early years at Esalen where Rolfing really got its start. The two books that she edited, *Ida Rolf Talks About Rolfing and Physical Reality* and *Remembering Ida Rolf*, are excellent references for learning more about Dr. Rolf and her thinking. I refer the interested reader to Dr. Rolf's main text, *Rolfing: The Integration of Human Structures*, published in 1977, which contains many excellent before-and-after photographs of people who have been Rolfed, and many anatomical drawings that greatly enhance any discussion of Rolfing.

What This Book Contains

I will briefly present the relationship of structure and function, how bodies become misaligned, and how Rolfing works to bring more order to structure. There will be discussion on working with shock and trauma, pathology and contraindications for Rolfing, as well as a section on the relationship of psychological and physical patterns of holding. We will also consider Rolfing as a tool for transformation and evolution in the last chapter. These chapters will be liberally sprinkled with stories, case histories, and interviews with some of my teachers.

This book will not exhaustively delve into the intricacies of human physiology, as there have already been many good books and papers written in that area. However, a basic knowledge of human anatomy and physiology is assumed. The reader who is unfamiliar with these areas will still profit from this book, as many of the concepts are explained briefly and appeal to commonsense. As best as I have been able, this book has been written from the heart, from my experiences, and from those of my clients and teachers.

My Background

Before I began my journey into Rolfing I had previously received a Bachelor of Science degree in physical education from Skidmore College in 1961. Even back in those days I had an abiding interest in the mind-body connection, and almost considered taking a major in psychology, but at that time this field felt too

With the soul, the body would have no form. Without the body, the soul would not have its required organs of sense through which it gains knowledge.

— THOMAS AQUINAS

left-brained for me. I taught physical education at the high school level and had an enjoyable time working with young people in the area of movement, dance, and sports. I received a Master of Science degree from the University of North Carolina at Greensboro in 1967 and moved to Tucson, Arizona in 1968 to teach at the University of Arizona, and later at a private Catholic school. I began to study Gestalt therapy and eventually received a Master of Education degree in counseling and guidance from the University of Arizona in Tucson.

This journey into Rolfing began for me in Tucson, where I met my first spiritual teacher, Swami Amar Jyoti, in 1976. It was he who gave me the suggestion to become a Rolfer, procured for me the interest-free loan to do the training, and sent me many clients over the years that I was with him. I had never expected to enter so deeply into the world of Rolfing, but once I began on that path, doors opened for me all along the way. I received my certification as a Rolfer from the Rolf Institute in 1978. My teachers from the auditing phase were Jan Sultan and Tom Wing, and for the practitioner phase, Emmett Hutchins and Tom Wing. My advanced training with Peter Melchior and Emmett Hutchins was completed in 1980. All four of these teachers were trained by Dr. Rolf.

Although I only met Ida Rolf once near the end of her life, my teachers brought her alive to me in their classes, and my class notes are filled with her quotes, received directly from my teachers. Many of the quotes in this book credited to Ida Rolf are from these class notes.

I dove headfirst into the Rolfing, returning to Tucson in 1978 to begin a private practice there. Within six months I had a full practice, and being the only Rolfer in the entire city and area, I could not defer to advanced practitioners when a problem arose with a client. I had to muddle on through on my own. As I was not trained in any other modality than Rolfing, I had to deepen my exploration of that craft in order to deal with challenges that

Ida Rolf has gone unrecognized as a major contributor to our understanding of the body...The whole idea that people could change and grow was suddenly thrust into our awareness. That is a monstrous paradigm change! Rolf stepped right into the middle of that with her technique, and people appropriated it [her technique] left and right, to grow in whatever ways they might have wanted to.

– JAN SULTAN

would come up in a session. Donna Jo Cross, a fellow Rolfer with whom I had trained, was beginning her practice in Scottsdale and we would speak by phone often to knock around questions we each had. We were both totally fired up by the work.

I continued to take classes and workshops: a six day workshop from Emmett Hutchins, another from Peter Melchior, advanced anatomy from Louis Schultz and Ron Thompson, perceptual training with Rosemary Feitis, and two workshops with Peter Levine in Somatic Experiencing®. After my advanced training, I was asked to be an assistant teacher, and for over seven years I taught classes with Emmett Hutchins, Peter Melchior, Stacy Mills, Tom Wing, and Nicholas French, all of whom had studied directly with Dr. Rolf. To be with these fine teachers in an assistantship relationship was a profound learning experience, and to share the work of Rolfing both as teacher and student allowed many opportunities for me to grow and expand both in myself and in the work.

In 1984 I moved to Boulder, Colorado, and became deeply involved with the Rolf Institute as the chair of the Admissions Committee, later serving on the Education Executive Committee, and the Board of Directors. I continued my apprenticeship with Emmett Hutchins during the years I lived in Boulder. Emmett and I often traded Rolfing sessions and I sometimes worked with him "four-handed," as we called it, with some of his clients. Needless to say, this was also a fabulous learning experience. My spiritual teacher had a center in Boulder and I was going there regularly for meditation and teachings.

The Split

During the 1980s the Rolf Institute began to strain at its moorings and eventually there was a split, allowing each side to grow in the direction they felt was true for them. In the following sections I will discuss that split. I will first briefly set the context regarding expansion of the original work, and then give a brief factual history of how the Guild for Structural Integration was reformed as a separate entity from the Rolf Institute for Structural Integration. It is important to introduce this at the beginning of this book, as it will make further reading clearer and will give an understanding of the ever broadening field of Structural Integration.

Expansion

It is inevitable that when a pioneer discovers or creates a new field of work that someday there will be branches of that work. New things will be discovered and different ways to accomplish goals will be tried. There will always be differing ideas about how the founder's work should be carried on, as well as how and if it should change as it grows. The overall challenge is how to maintain the good name established by the founder, especially when her particular ideas and discoveries became popular. Specifically, questions to be considered will be: Does one form an organization? Should it be non-profit? Should one try to obtain a service mark? How does one protect the service mark? How do you define what it is you are protecting?

Some examples of pioneers in the healing arts field would be Moshe Feldenkrais of The Feldenkrais Method®, Dr. Andrew Taylor Still of Osteopathy, Marion Rosen of the Rosen Method, Joseph H. Pilates of the Pilates Method, and of course Dr. Ida P. Rolf of Rolfing. A quick glance on the Internet under these names will show you the varying ways that each method has unfolded.

Osteopathy is a good example of how a powerful discovery unfolded through the years and influenced many other pioneers, including Dr. Rolf. Dr. Andrew Taylor Still, considered the founder of osteopathy, formed the American School of Osteopathy in 1892; now known as the Kirksville College of Osteopathic Medicine. In the early 1900s, Dr. William G. Sutherland, an osteopathic physician, discovered the intrinsic movement of the bones of the skull and the cranial rhythm. He was the founder of what we know today as cranial osteopathy, which is a branch of practice for Doctors of Osteopathy (D.O.s). Later on, Dr. John E. Upledger, also an osteopathic physician, pioneered and developed craniosacral therapy or CST. He later formed the Upledger Institute and made CST training available for the first time to non-physicians. Michael Shea, originally a Rolfer, then developed Biodynamic Craniosacral Therapy which incorporated not only craniosacral therapy, but also influences from Charlotte Selver, William Sutherland, Carl Jung, Marie Louise Von Franz, Elsa Gindler, Wilhelm Reich, Ida Rolf, Fritz Perls, and Ken Wilber.

A wonderful piece in Feitis's book, *Ida Rolf Talks*, concerns this early history of osteopathy and Dr. Rolf's part in it. Dr. Rolf says: "Dr. Still somehow or other got the notion that function had something to do with structure, had some dependence on structure, and that by altering structure he could alter function. That is the same premise that we are operating on today."[2] Feitis goes on: "The osteopathic concept as it was originally formulated by Dr. Still, had a big, a wide understanding of the use of soft tissue. He was the first man who expressed the idea that not only does structure determine function, but that it is possible to change function by changing structure."[3]

So we could say that both Dr. Rolf and Dr. Sutherland were influenced by Dr. Still's idea of the relationship between structure and function. Dr. Rolf was often frustrated in trying to teach her method of working with structure and function, however, and with trying to get her students to stick with the method. Feitis quotes her as follows:

When you have a new idea and you want to get it across, you'd better be well armed with a sledgehammer and a chisel in order to make a hole in your listeners' skulls. When they think they understand, they have perceived just one essential point of it. But you have the whole of it and to you it is so obvious.[4]

The original osteopaths were comparable to Rolfers. But then every student got his little ego trip going and every little ego tripper knew that he knew a little more than the old boy, so they tried a little something new. So you thin it and you dilute it and you take it off its course. When you get through you have something different going...If I can keep you people together and out of your ego trip until we get from here to there, we'll be that much better off. Hang together at this point in your thinking; don't try improvements just now. Otherwise you go off on tangents. There are improvements possible, I'm sure, but wait a little.[5]

You can always tell something about how good a Rolfer is by how many supplementary techniques he'll try to use. I'm not saying that Rolfing is the be-all and end-all of existence. I don't think that it is. I don't think it's the last word, but I do think that if you took every one of the concepts we've used and expanded them in the right direction, you'd have something that is. If you stay with this one set of ideas you will get the job done.[6]

Today, twenty-five or thirty years later, there are approximately twelve schools that teach some aspects of Dr. Rolf's Ten-Session Series Recipe. Tom Myers in his article entitled "Developments of Ida Rolf's Recipe" makes some clear general statements about where we are at present regarding the terms "Rolfing" and "Structural Integration" or SI.

While every attempt has been made to get the facts straight, there is much debate within the SI community as to which key concepts are primary, the exact intent of Ida Rolf when

Great spirits have always encountered violent opposition from mediocre minds.
— ALBERT EINSTEIN

contradictory statements appear in the record, as well as to the actual application and scope of practice of SI...In the inevitable fractures and resultant legal battles which followed Dr. Rolf's death, the term "Rolfing" became a registered service mark of the Rolf Institute, which is now one of perhaps a dozen schools of SI. Therefore, "Structural Integration," the last of several of Dr. Rolf's original names for her work, is becoming the generic designation for this type of manipulative approach.[7]

Brief History of the Split

As in all history there is a story that unfolds that is based in part on the memory of the people who participated at the time. The information that follows is based on the facts I was able to gather from an interview with Rosemary Feitis, D.O., an advanced Rolfer, who was Dr. Rolf's secretary from 1968 to 1972, and an unrecorded interview with Richard Stenstadvold, Executive Director of the Rolf Institute from 1972-1988, and President of the Guild for Structural Integration (GSI), 1988 to present. A phone interview with Karna Knapp of the Rolf Institute provided information regarding dates and documents.

In the early years of Esalen Institute in Big Sur, California, Dr. Rolf would come to Esalen in the summers and teach classes. In the mid 1960s, Dr. Rolf and her practitioners formed the original Guild for Structural Integration – born out of the same ideology as the Guild of Hands, a group of artisans from Esalen that included Peter Melchior. Although the Guild was not a legally created organization, it served as a way to help organize Dr. Rolf's students. In the early 1970s the unincorporated Guild for Structural Integration was re-formed legally as The Rolf Institute of Structural Integration®. In 1972, at Dr. Rolf's request, Richard Stenstadvold, who was previously the business manager for

Our bodies are our gardens – our wills are our gardeners.
— WILLIAM SHAKESPEARE

Adolph's Food Products and had met Dr. Rolf through Emmett
Hutchins, agreed to become the business manager for this newly
formed Rolf organization. Later on, after the Rolf Institute had
become incorporated, the term "Rolfing" was registered with the
U.S. patent office. To quote from the 2003/2004 catalog of the
Rolf Institute: "In 1979, the United States Patent Office granted
service mark rights for the word Rolfing to the Rolf Institute of
Structural Integration, distinguishing the Rolfing brand from all
other forms of structural integration."[8]

After Dr. Rolf's passing in 1979, Richard continued on as
Executive Director of the Rolf Institute. In 1988, Richard, along
with some of the senior faculty and staff left the Rolf Institute.
Richard then re-formed the original Guild for Structural
Integration, incorporating it as a non-profit institution. Emmett
Hutchins taught the first Structural Integration class for the Guild
for Structural Integration (GSI) in 1990; Stacey Mills taught the
second class for GSI and soon after both Emmett and Stacey left
the Rolf Institute. Peter Melchior also left the Rolf Institute and
began teaching for GSI. Since that time some Rolfers have left the
Rolf Institute and joined GSI, some have stayed with the Rolf
Institute, and some remain members of both organizations. I
remain a member of both organizations.

In the meantime, other schools formed that included
Structural Integration in their curricula. At present there are about
ten such schools other than GSI and The Rolf Institute. Dr. Rolf's
original name for her work was Structural Integration. It later
came to be known as Rolfing. Since the split in the Rolf Institute,
Structural Integration has become the generic name for Rolfing. I
have used the words Rolfing and Structural Integration inter-
changeably in this book. However, at present, the two words are no
longer necessarily interchangeable in meaning. The Rolf Institute
owns the service mark to the word "Rolfing" and thus Emmett and

Peter, who are no longer members of the Rolf Institute, may not legally call their work other than the Ida Rolf Method of Structural Integration, or just Structural Integration.

Of Dr. Rolf's first teachers who trained directly with her, three are teaching at the Guild for Structural Integration: Emmett Hutchins, Peter Melchior, and Neal Powers. (Stacey Mills taught for GSI until her passing.) Three presently teach at the Rolf Institute: Jan Sultan, Michael Salveson, and Jim Asher. Tom Wing continues to Rolf but is no longer teaching.

I was on the Board at the time of the split and it was a tremendous challenge to try to serve in an open, non-judgmental way when friends and people close to me were feeling a lot of pain and upset. My spiritual teacher's center became a life raft for me to float on and come back to each day, enabling me a level of detachment in order to do my job as a board member during this crisis.

My Own Work Continues

Around 1986 I met a dancer and artist named Paul Oertel. His wife Nancy Spanier had a dance company, all of whom were Rolfed by Emmett Hutchins. Together we made many deep explorations of the relationship of Rolfing and how it opened the way for authentic expression. Paul and I worked together in his studio for an hour a week and, over an eight-year period, we explored authentic movement, expression of feeling in art, issues of the client-therapist relationship, and other areas too numerous to mention. He is one of the most brilliant people I have ever met in terms of his lifelong study of opening one to one's deep and true potential for authentic expression. From him I learned about "the discipline of freedom" and what a powerful healing-tool such artistic expression can be.

After the split of the Rolf Institute and the formation of the Guild for Structural Integration, I somewhat retreated into the "magic box" of my Rolfing room. By 1993 I knew clearly that my work and time in Boulder was over. I had left my spiritual teacher's ashram in 1993, and in 1994 I moved back to live with my mother on a large family property in Vermont. My dad had died in 1991, so my mom had been living there alone. For the next eight years I maintained a good Rolfing practice, enjoying "the farm" as we called it. I had a huge organic garden on my dad's garden site and got very intrigued with nature spirits and the energy of the land. In 2002 we had to sell the property, and in August of 2003 my mother died. Things were complete now in Vermont and my restless urge to come home once again to Arizona that had been brewing over the last three years was free to be realized.

I had thought of going back to Tucson where I had so many friends, but I felt it was too hot and too big. I spent the winter of 2001 finding out everything I could about a place that seemed to attract me – Prescott, Arizona. That spring I came out and spent a week in Prescott and left knowing that this would be my next home. After the sale of our Vermont property was complete, I moved to Prescott to begin my Rolfing practice anew again. This time I really didn't know anyone except one person I knew from long back in Tucson who had just moved here too. I began putting cards and flyers around and soon spirit was to lead me once again in a direction I never would have dreamed. The first person to come to me for Rolfing was part of a spiritual community here in Prescott. In searching for a good yoga class, I landed at Prescott Yoga with teacher Christina Sell, also a member of this spiritual community led by Lee Lozowick. I began reading his books and found a deep resonance with his teachings. In the course of becoming involved with his community I was invited to write a book on Rolfing. And so I have been given a wonderful opportunity to take this Rolfing journey again, through this book, and to share with my colleagues in the healing arts world a bit about this work that has been a part of my life these twenty-seven years.

I live in company with a body, a silent companion, exacting and eternal.
– EUGENE DELACROIX

In the interviews with my Rolfing teachers I did not always ask each of them exactly the same question in the same way, so each has responded in different depths. The interviews were actually quite spontaneous and went in many directions based on what was unfolding at the time. Again, I am sure that each of my Rolf teachers could write his own book from his own perspective, so the quotes from them in this book are just to give a taste of each.

I have endeavored to the best of my ability through the lens of my own perception and my experience to represent what each of my teachers has taught. Whatever comes out in my words is riding on my deep deep appreciation and love for them and all they have given me, not only their passion for Rolfing, but also their very being. Rolfing is a way of life, as each of my teachers have often said. We are all a part of Dr. Rolf's experiment in human evolution and I am proud to be involved in such an endeavor.

Endnotes, Introduction

[1] The word "Rolfing" is a service mark of the Rolf Institute of Structural Integration, Boulder, Colorado.
[2] Feitis, Rosemary, Editor. *Ida Rolf Talks About Rolfing and Physical Reality.* New York, New York: Harper and Row, 1978, 165.
[3] Ibid., 166.
[4] Ibid., 167.
[5] Ibid., 170.
[6] Ibid., 178.
[7] Myers, Tom. "Developments In Ida Rolf's Recipe." *2004 Yearbook of Structural Integration.* Missoula, Montana: International Association of Structural Integrators, 2004, 16.
[8] *Rolf Institute Educational Catalog 2003-2004.* Boulder, Colorado: The Rolf Institute, 2.

Part I

The Founder

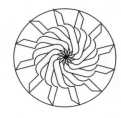

1
Dr. Ida P. Rolf, 1896-1979
Pioneer, Scientist, Teacher, Mystic

She sits in the center of a room, a commanding presence with snow-white hair pulled up onto her head and held in place with many combs. A fresh flower is pinned in her hair. Her students sit around her, notebooks in hand, while a small boy of about eleven years stands up on the plywood Rolfing table. She looks like the classic sweet old grandmother, but as someone once put it, "Dr. Rolf is a little old white-haired Sherman tank." She is asking her students what they see, prodding them, demanding answers to her questions and then interacting with each as they speak. The camera is often at odd angles as it is most likely on a tripod with little room to move.

I am watching an archival video of Dr. Ida P. Rolf, founder and developer of the system called Structural Integration, better known as Rolfing. This video is called "The Boy Logan Series,"[1] which was probably filmed in 1971/1972 when Dr. Rolf was seventy-six years of age. Traffic roars by somewhere outside, yet the audio picks up her voice – a voice with a slight New York accent; a voice that is clearly heard by all as she talks in her normal tone. She speaks slowly and with emphasis. There is no hesitation. Here is a person who knows what she wants to say.

Later in the program, as Dr. Rolf begins to work directly on Logan, the camera zooms in on her hands. I am struck by how gnarled they are. The knuckles of the first finger are permanently bent and the other fingers are slanted and twisted from her years of hard work – changing tissue in hundreds of bodies using nothing but her hands, knuckles, and an occasional elbow. She wears a wedding ring and watch on her left hand and her glasses dangle from her neck on a strap. Her touch is extremely specific. She knows exactly what she wants to change. Her vision is beyond remarkable. She's working deeply in Logan's tissue, yet he is not flinching or drawing back. Dr. Rolf is totally direct and real with no pretense. Perhaps that is one reason why Logan is so cooperative, both in allowing Dr. Rolf to work on him and in his willingness to stand and walk and be viewed by the class as she instructs her students in learning to see structure.

When she [Ida] put her hands on you, you just knew that her hands had the ability to connect in a way that could interact with your body and get it to change. What fascinated me was watching her hands working like a sculptor, almost.
— HADIDJAH LAMAS, *REMEMBERING IDA ROLF*, 13.

In this particular video Dr. Rolf is demonstrating the second hour in the Ten-Series "Recipe" (*see* Chapter 5 for more information on the Ten Series). In this hour, Dr. Rolf is considering the base of support for the body and is paying particular attention to Logan's feet and lower legs. She begins to work in a specific and focused way on the retinaculum just above Logan's left ankle. After about three moves in just a few minutes, she asks Logan to flex his ankle again. Even in this old funky video I can immediately see the dramatic change in this simple movement. Unexpected tears spring to my eyes and I find myself, a Rolfer of twenty-seven years, asking, "How did she *do* that?"

How did Dr. Ida Rolf come to this point in her life where she is teaching a class about the work that she spent most of her life developing? In 1977 Dr. Rolf was in her eighty-first year. The Rolf Institute had been formed in 1971/1972 in Boulder, Colorado, with Richard Stenstadvold as executive director. In 1977, the book *Rolfing: The Integration of Human Structures* was published. It is "the major written statement of Ida P. Rolf's scholastic and experiential investigation into the direct intervention with the evolution of the human species."[2] She had trained approximately 150 actively-practicing Rolfers, and Lisa Connolly in her May 1977 article in *Human Behavior* estimated, in an interview with Dr. Rolf, that approximately 55,000 people in the U.S., Mexico, France, The Netherlands, Canada, England, Germany, Israel, and India had been Rolfed.[3] Quite an accomplishment for one lifetime!

In the introduction to *Ida Rolf Talks About Rolfing and Physical Reality*, Rosemary Feitis, the editor, writes an engaging history of Dr. Rolf's early years. According to Feitis:

> IPR was born in New York in 1896 and grew up in the Bronx. She attended Barnard College, graduating in 1916 in the middle of World War I. At that time, with young men fighting in Europe, the supply of qualified technical personnel in so many fields was pre-empted, and so she was given a unique opportunity for a woman of that time. She was hired by Rockefeller Institute (now Rockefeller University) in New York City, and allowed to continue her education while working there. She received a Ph.D. in biological chemistry from the College of Physicians and Surgeons of Columbia University and continued at Rockefeller, eventually gaining the rank of associate.[4]

The catalog of the Guild for Structural Integration states that: "In 1927, she took a leave of absence from her work to study mathematics and atomic physics at the Swiss Technical University in Zurich. During this time she also studied homeopathic medicine in Geneva."[5]

When Ida Rolf returned from Geneva, she spent much of the 1930s exploring osteopathy, chiropractic medicine, yoga, the Alexander technique and Korzybski's work on states of consciousness. In working with her own personal and family health challenges, she had not found the answers she sought in the medical field and thus was drawn to these more holistic methods.

Dr. Rolf had a tremendous breadth of education for a woman growing up in the 1920s during World War I. Her library contained a wide variety of medical dictionaries as well as books by Reich, Bates, C.W. Leadbeater, Emmanuel Swedenborg, and many others from a great variety of sources. When perusing her archival library at The Rolf Institute, I also noticed books such as *The Dramatic Universe* by J. G. Bennett, *To Touch Infinity* by Salisbury, and *The God of the Witches* by Murray. She was obviously a woman with a brilliant and probing mind as well as a force of will and an inner confidence that allowed her to get away with the audacity of putting her hands into a person's connective tissue with the intent to change his or her structure.

Dr. Rolf was primarily a scientist and wanted her work clearly grounded in the reality of physics, biology, and chemistry. Yet many of her breakthroughs came intuitively and were not always easily explained through the science available at the time. Within the last ten years, and with the development of the electron microscope and other scientific tools along with new discoveries in Quantum physics, many of her intuitive insights can now be examined in new ways. She hoped that Rolfing would be accepted by the scientific and medical world, though research in Rolfing was difficult to do and proved minimal at best. (*See* Chapter 12, *Research*.) One of her key premises was that a body could actually *change*, and for the better – a concept that was not generally held until some of the breakthroughs of the Human Potential Movement that came in the 1960s. Dr. Rolf would say that if you wanted a different result you must start with a different premise. In a 1974 lecture she declared: "One of the premises that will lead you further is the recognition that human beings are dynamic units. They are energy units; they are movement units; they are summations of energy units."[6]

Dr. Rolf was challenging the basic Aristotelian premises that bodies begin, grow, mature, deteriorate, and die, and that other than that cannot be changed. She was introducing in her teaching and her work that by changing one part of a person, everything else that was connected to that part would also change. In an article written in 1962, she again noted the idea that physical structure is deeply related to human behavior: "Since it seems demonstrable that man's outer world is a projection of that which is within, is it not possible that some of the problems of our times might be resolved by examining the man himself, his physical being, his body."[7]

Perhaps the most unique contribution of Dr. Rolf's thinking was the sense that the human being was organized around a vertical line, and lived in an environment of a gravitational field. In a small article titled *Rolfing: The Vertical Experiential Side to Human Potential*, put out by the Rolf Institute in 1977, she mused about this possibility:

If any thing is sacred, the human body is sacred.
– WALT WHITMAN

What happens when soft tissue and related bone structure actually function in the positions in space which their architectural design suggests as most appropriate and which contributes most effectively to establishing the vertical? The vertical in man's structure is the outcome of his proprioceptive, sensory appreciation of the gravity pull of the earth. Whether consciously or unconsciously, he feels this pull and responds to it. This is a subtle concept: the intellectual formulation arises out of the sensory awareness. Man's appreciation of the vertical evolves from his sense of the gravity pull of the earth.[8]

This same article begins with a bold statement of her interest in changing structure:

First let me reiterate what I have often said before: I as an individual, am not primarily interested in the relief of symptoms, either physical or mental. To hear Rolfees tell of their "wonderful," "unbelievable," symptom alleviation, it's hard not to accept this assessment as a goal. However, I am interested in human potential, and human potential per se neither includes nor excludes the palliation of symptoms.[9]

Dr. Rolf also had a deep inner spiritual and metaphysical side, but she kept this mostly to herself. Occasionally she would experiment with and briefly discuss human energy fields as she did in the advanced Rolfing class with Dr. Brugh Joy at Sky Hi Ranch in 1977. Videos of that class show some of the students with their hands off the body feeling for energy, particularly the energy coming off the top of the head after a session of Rolfing. Each of the four teachers whom I interviewed mentioned this spiritual/metaphysical leaning of Dr. Rolf's, noting particularly that they could feel that she had a special energy about her.

Peter Melchior

She had a power that was just hard to believe. I mean it wasn't pushing, it wasn't physical strength, it was just this energy. It was quite extraordinary, and my energy responded to it in extraordinary ways…Ida Rolf was a great admirer of Gurdjieff's work and she believed with him that man was not finished; that evolution was finished as an unconscious process; [but] that the next step would take conscious participation.[10]

Jan Sultan

I think she [Dr. Rolf] was caught in a double bind. She had the scientific training, and that made her want to put [Rolfing] on the map as a repeatable, dependable modality,

Ida did not want us to work with sick people. She wanted us to work with healthy people. She wanted Rolfing to further healthy people on their evolutionary path. It was dangerous to work with sick people – we'd get sued and the AMA would get after us…very scary. There was a city ordinance in Los Angeles that women masseuses had to work only on women. You could get thrown in jail for working on a man – and vice versa.
– HADIDJAH LAMAS,
REMEMBERING IDA
ROLF, 11.

but she had her own metaphysics – her whole involvement with Korzybski and J.G. Bennett. [Bennett was a prominent leader of the Gurdjieff work in London. She often spent summers in England as his guest and he arranged groups to see her demonstrations.[11]] In her lectures she would often digress into these subjects, but then would say that unless you can demonstrate what you are talking about, keep your metaphysics to yourself.[12]

Emmett Hutchins

She was an infinitely logical being and she never depended on metaphysics for anything – not to prove her work or even to verify her work. She did try to use it with an aura reader in the UCLA project, but she never depended on anything but basic physics and pure simple logic to describe her work, and never needed to. But privately, and in some classes, especially classes where she had people who didn't want to hear that kind of thing, she would speak of metaphysical ideas. One of her goals seemed to have been to disturb everybody's complacency, and their little universe, and how they thought it worked. So, if she got a hold of a class of physicists and intellectuals, then she would spring all her metaphysical stuff on them because she knew that would blow them away. But most of the time she didn't talk about it at all.[13]

Tom Wing

She was well versed in metaphysics. In terms of her teaching work I think she was very careful about that. She would say to people, "Well, metaphysics is just physics that hasn't been discovered yet or proved yet,"…and then she would also say, "You work on the physics and let the metaphysics take care of themselves." To me, one of the seminal statements she made one time, [was]: "I believe a man has many bodies, a physical body, a spiritual body," she named a couple of others – energy body…She said, "and probably one hundred others we don't have names for yet. Furthermore I believe that these are interconnected and to affect one affects them all." She said, "So I choose to get my hands on what I can get my hands on and change that, knowing that it doesn't stop there." She was open to those considerations but not open to talking about them.[14]

I was fascinated by Ida's hands. They were unusual. It was the kind of contact they had. She was really in charge of that tissue. She really knew. People would ask her, "What are you doing? How do you know what to do?" She would answer, "My hands tell me what to do."

– HADIDJAH LAMAS,
REMEMBERING IDA
ROLF, 13.

And get her hands on people she did! All through the 1940s and 50s she worked with a great variety of people, experimenting and developing her work. She taught all over the country – in Texas, Los Angeles, Chicago – as well as in England. But most of this teaching was to chiropractors and osteopaths who used her work as an adjunct to their own work. They used her techniques but not her premises. She wanted Rolfing to be accepted as a separate body of work and knowledge. However, these professionals were licensed to touch, well educated in the physical sciences, and had established practices of their own. The people Dr. Rolf was to run into later at Esalen, people who were to become her core group of teachers, had little or no training in the sciences. They were required to study anatomy and physiology and obtain a massage license in order to practice as Rolfers. Nevertheless, she continued working wherever she could and continued to capture the attention of all she touched.

Amazingly, Dr. Rolf was developing a way in which you could use your hands to actually change the placement of connective tissue around bones and joints so that the individual had improved physiological and psychological functioning, as well as freer movement and better posture. The means by which she could reliably teach this to others and still gain repeatable results while remaining within safe boundaries was what later came to be called Ida Rolf's

"Recipe" or the Ten-Session Series of Rolfing. When questioned about how she came up with this, Dr. Rolf is vague, but there is a certain sharpness in the following quote from *Ida Rolf Talks*:

> ...when you start, you start with a couple of broken sticks if that's all you can find. People today don't understand that. When you start from zero, you start from zero, and by God you work. You put your back in it, and your head in it, and you don't give any attention to anything else.[15]

Both Melchior and Wing expressed in their interviews that they felt as though Dr. Rolf had been gifted with a vision of the whole process and then worked to refine it. Like the scientist who discovered the chemical benzene chain while in a moment of deep relaxation, Dr. Rolf may have had a breakthrough kind of perception in discovering the Ten Series. But, if this was indeed true, she was only rewarded with such an experience after years and years of hard work.

1960s and 1970s – Meetings with a Remarkable Woman

Around the year 1965 (dates vary in different reports but it was in the mid-1960s), Dr. Rolf got a big break. She was invited to come to Esalen Institute in Big Sur, California to do some Rolfing with Fritz Perls (the founder of Gestalt therapy) who was suffering from heart trouble. The 1960s were times of explosive changes rippling through the culture – the protests and marches against the Vietnam War; Students for a Democratic Society; the Black Panthers; The Beatles; Indian gurus; Ram Dass; the drug culture; hippies; civil rights marches; and Martin Luther King. A similar movement of change was going on at Esalen on the California coast, which was a primary showcase for new and cutting-edge work in the human potential movement.

Will Schutz, Abraham Maslow, Wilhelm Reich, Stanislov Grof, as well as Fritz Perls, were exploring the realm of the interrelationship of mind/body/spirit in groundbreaking ways. Dr. Rolf was right in the middle of this as the only one approaching such changes directly from the organization of physical structure. She had little respect for psychology, but as she came to know Fritz Perls and his Gestalt therapy, and he came to experience her work by being Rolfed by her, and later sending many of his students to get Rolfed, the two of them gained quite a mutual respect for each other.

Around this same time, Peter Melchior was living at Esalen, working on the staff, and taking seminars from Fritz Perls. Peter describes his first meeting with Dr. Rolf as follows:

I remember we were sitting in Fritz's house. We'd lie on the floor and listen to Beethoven's violin concerto – that was part of the training [he chuckles]. And then one day there was this presence at the door, you know – wham, like Count Dracula! It was Ida, and she immediately just walked into the room and said, "Take off your shirt old man," and we thought *who the hell is this*? Nobody tells Fritz Perls to take off his shirt! And meekly he gets up and starts taking off his shirt. Apparently he'd heard of her or something. [Dorothy Nolte had given him about three Rolfing sessions and then suggested he should really go see Dr. Rolf.] This is getting stranger and stranger, and so she takes a look at him standing there with his shirt off and she turns to me and she says, 'Well no wonder the man's having heart attacks. Look at the left side of his chest. It's all caved in! Why haven't you done something about this?" I said, "I'm an English major. What the hell am I supposed to do about it?" [Laughter] So she says "Pshaw," you know, and goes on working on him – works for about forty-five minutes. He gets up; he says, "I feel better." And I said, "Oh come on!" He says, "No, no, no I really feel better."

She sticks around for a little over a month and she works on him probably twelve sessions over the time she's there and he just keeps getting better and better and better. Understand, this is a guy who has had two major cardiac festivals and he's smoking four packs of Kents a day...somebody would have to take him [Fritz] to the baths and back when he wanted to go. [Down at the hot spring baths was the place Dr. Rolf was working.] It would take all day because coming back up the hill was like [Fritz would take] four steps and...(Peter breathes hard), you know. By the time [he's] gotten six or seven sessions he's striding up the hill next to me. I'm like, "What the hell is happening here?" I've never seen anything like this in my life![16]

Emmett Hutchins was working for Boeing as an engineering aide. His job was to program the large computer they had back in the late 1950s. In those days, no one knew how to run those first computers except the engineers who had designed them. Emmett became one of the few who understood how to work these huge computers. He too first ran into Rolfing in California, but not at Esalen. In the early 1960s, when Emmett was around thirty-two or thirty-three, he was visiting a friend and heard about a woman who had had some amazing results from Rolfing, including getting some arches in her feet. Emmett elaborated:

I'd always had flat feet, and my father had made me feel like it was a personality flaw, which he was probably pretty close to being accurate about. But, back in those days, such a thing sounded pretty quirky...When I heard of this woman who could "do arches" I went over, and that was Hadijah

[T]his very body that we have, that's sitting right here right now... with its aches and its pleasures...is exactly what we need to be fully human, fully awake, fully alive.
    – PEMA CHÖDRUN

Fielding, who I think only met Ida Rolf once. She was a practitioner trained by Stacey Mills, because Ida's original plan for getting practitioners was from the "old school" – you had the master and the adepts, and the adepts picked another student to pass on the training to. So Stacey, who was Ida's student, had picked Hadijah Fielding, who lived in California, to be one of her students. I went there and I asked her questions the whole time. I was thirty-four years old and I had a pain in my back constantly so I was interested in getting my feet and the pain in my back fixed.

I didn't notice that my arches got much better in the Ten Sessions, but I did feel like she had gotten to me, and changed me in many ways, and my back pain had changed. It hadn't gone away but it had changed, and it would be better for awhile after she worked on me.

I asked Hadijah all these questions, and she never answered any of them because she did all of her work as a part of her spiritual discipline and so she never uttered a word. We'd work on the floor, and she never uttered a word once I lay down…A year and a half after I had finished my tenth hour she called me one evening and said, "Do you remember those questions you used to ask me?" I was surprised she'd even remembered, because she had never acknowledged that I even had asked her a question. I said, "Well, some of them." And she said, "Well, Dr. Rolf is in town and she's teaching a class and the class started this morning and I have her phone number and maybe you'd like to call her and see if you can ask *her* some of those questions."

I called her [Dr. Rolf] up and she wanted to know who I was and how I got her number. I told her that Hadijah had told me that she was starting a class, and then asked, "Maybe I could just join it and audit in your class?"

She said to me, "Oh absolutely not. All the basics of the class have been done. The class is well started and there's just no way you can catch up now," and on and on.

I started to hang up and then she said, "Now don't ring off yet." She started chatting and asked me if I'd ever taught anybody anything, and a bunch of other things. Finally, just before she hung up, she said, "Well, how about you just show up in the morning about 8:00 AM," and she gave me her room number at the Beverly Hills Sands, and then, click. She didn't say goodbye or anything. I later learned that she never said goodbye on the phone. When her business was done she wasn't there anymore.[17]

The next morning I walked in early, as I usually do, and the door was ajar on this motel room. I later learned that nobody knew she was having a class there. It was just her motel room. I walked in and there was an old lady with a big cape on bending over a cot in the kitchenette part of this place, and she was doing something. A woman was lying on the cot, and at the foot of the bed was another woman with her hands about eight inches from the feet of the woman on the bed, and she was telling Ida, "No, it's a little on the left, it's a little on the right." She was feeling something in her space and her hands were about eight inches off the feet. There was a wire running from under the patient. She was lying on an aluminum plate and this wire ran under the cot and wrapped around the faucet in the kitchen.

My impression was that I'd walked in on something just totally other worldly; something that I had no idea about. I had no way to anticipate what was going on.[18]

At the time, Emmett had no intention of going on to train to become a Rolfer, but Dr. Rolf had other plans for him.

There was an "esoteric" part of Rolfing in the 1950's. The early Rolfers used to use foot plates — metal plates on the feet — to help pull the energy releases out during the session. By the time I came on the scene Ida had abandoned that, but if there was someone available they would hold the client's feet to help the energy release. In my early practice, we would have the client hold a small empty juice can that had been grounded with a wire to facilitate releasing.
– HADIDJAH LAMAS,
REMEMBERING IDA
ROLF, 9.

At the end of the class (three or four months later) Ida said, "Well, I suppose we'll be seeing you up at Big Sur." And I said, "Oh, I don't think so," because I still had not thought about doing it as a living. I was only interested in what would happen to me. (She worked on me three times during the class when I audited.)

The next day, when I talked to her, I thought…well, maybe I'll get her goat, and so I said, "You know, Ida, I'm not really interested in helping people." And she looked at me and she said, "Oh? What *are* you interested in?"

I said, "I'm really interested in my own spiritual evolution, my own mystical awakening. I want to meet the Great White Brotherhood." I was trying to get her to tell me to go somewhere else or something.

Wheresoever you go, go with all your heart.
    – CONFUCIUS

She looked at me and said, "I don't know how to introduce you to those boys, but I do know that if you spend enough time" and she pointed down to the floor where we work [doing Rolfing in those days], "if you spend enough time down there, when they're ready to find you they will."

With that kind of a challenge you can't say no, even if you don't believe it. I decided to go to the class in Big Sur.[19]

A few years later, around 1968, Jan Sultan entered the picture. At the time he was dividing his time between working in the building trade – doing masonry work, rough carpentry and framing – and going to sea as an ordinary seaman and engine room wiper, as he also had a merchant seaman's license. Jan explained: "Well I actually had some friends who were living at Esalen. I was on an oceanographic survey that was based in Monterey. I would go down to Big Sur to socialize and play, and I had some friends who had contacted Dr. Rolf at Esalen. In the course of conversation I began to think it would be an interesting venue for me to try." Dr. Rolf gave Jan his first eight sessions and then Peter Melchior, who had just trained with Ida, completed the Ten Series with Jan.[20]

In the meantime, Tom Wing was finishing his masters degree in library science and, in 1970, he got a job at Prescott College in Prescott, Arizona as assistant librarian. Prescott College was at that time (and remains) an experimental college with courses and explorations in the humanities. Tom began taking a dance class there from Heather Wing, who had been Rolfed in California. She talked up Rolfing and arranged for a Rolfer to come to Prescott from California.

Tom signed up to be Rolfed. He had a most painful experience getting the first session from the Rolfer, but the changes in his breathing were so dramatic that he decided to continue. "After the second session I started to be able to wiggle my toes and that was it. It was like…O.K., this is wild and crazy, and an unusual and exciting thing." He finished his Ten Series with Jan Sultan, who by then had been trained as a Rolfer. The long and the short of it was that Tom became impassioned with the work and even though he had no background in the sciences, he decided he wanted to train to become a Rolfer. In those days the admissions "committee" consisted of Dr. Rolf alone. Tom recalled his first meeting with Dr. Rolf in her apartment on Riverside Drive in New York City:[21]

I get to the door…and Rosemary [Dr. Rolf's secretary at the time] opens the door and I walk in. There's this long room with Ida at the far corner sitting in a chair with a lap desk. She looks up from her lap desk across the room at me standing in the doorway and starts shrieking, as Ida could, "No! No! No! Why do all you little people think you can be Rolfers?" Rosemary brought me in and Ida spent the next few minutes just telling me all the ways in which I was totally unacceptable and culminating with the wonderful:

"Besides, you're an imploded mesomorph. You can't be a Rolfer that way."

At that point I had to say something. So I said, "What does that mean, an imploded mesomorph?"

"What that means is that all of your energy...starts out but it doesn't get out. Before it gets out it turns back on itself, so you don't put any energy out of your system whatsoever. You just circulate it inside. You are imploded. You've got to learn how to turn your energy around because you can't do Rolfing with your energy doing that."[22]

What an introduction! But Wing's story is significant. Evidently Rolfing had deeply affected him, because he went on to take the necessary courses and work through Arica® training to turn his energy around. He trained as a Rolfer two years later.

Intrigued by the stories of how my teachers first met Dr. Rolf, and thoroughly impressed by the perseverance and focus they each demonstrated in order to train in Rolfing with Dr. Rolf, I asked them, *What was the most profound and lasting concept, introduced by Dr. Rolf, that captivated you?*

Peter

The idea that the situation could be changed! She said flat out: "There's no situation in the human body that I've ever seen that hasn't been able to be affected in some way." As far as I was concerned you got issued a body and that was it, and if you didn't like it, too bad. That's what changed for me in my first session of Rolfing. "Oh my God, this is a lot more mutable than that. This is a whole different thing," I thought.[23]

Emmett

The "Line" (*see* Chapter 4) – that's where the weightlessness comes from…It's just the very basic fact that Mother Earth cannot lift me up in the air any harder than I am willing to give weight to her. You become weightless because you give it all up. You put it all down. If you throw it all down you don't feel it anymore, because then it is supported by the earth. I'm still trying to get all my weight into the earth. The more I do that, and the better my feet get, the more I get rid of the scar tissue from the early traumas in my life, the lighter I get. Really, many times I have the feeling of weighing almost nothing in space. Certainly when I am meditating I can get to that place. I'm trying to get to that place while I'm walking down the street. So far that hasn't happened, but it's approaching. After all, it's a path.

I have no requirement that these things ever happen to me…It's been a wonderful path, and it doesn't make any difference if I ever achieve some of those things. I think your goals *ought to be* unrealizable, or you're going to get there too soon. So, I've chosen goals that I know I'm not going to get to too soon, maybe never at all. To me that's very exciting. "It's not the getting there it's the going there," as many many many people have said, but it's really true…I am at the place where I…feel like just putting my Line in every day brings on a new layer of awareness and then something new happens every single day whether anybody works with me or not.[24]

Jan

First, it was the impact on my structure – the initial opening of my lungs; and then I read her book *Gravity*, the little booklet she had out at the time, and gravity made sense

Dance as if no one were watching, sing as if no one were listening, and live every day as if it were your last.

– IRISH PROVERB

to me because I was a builder: if you don't get things stacked they are not stable.

The whole idea that people could change and grow was suddenly thrust into our awareness. I'm in a Spanish culture here where I live, and they do not have the idea that people can change and grow. That is a monstrous paradigm change. Rolf stepped right into the middle of that with her technique and people appropriated it left and right to grow in whatever ways they might have wanted to.

She said all these things in the body are in relationship. You can't affect one without affecting everything else, so a comprehensive approach was called for...And that leads you right into personality, psychology, the orientation of the individual to their growth – you know spiritually and maturing, being able to make finer and finer distinctions was a function of being able to language your perception differently.[25]

Health of body and mind is a great blessing, if we can bear it.

– JOHN HENRY CARDINAL NEWMAN

Tom

I started clearing stuff out of my lungs – I had twenty years of chronic bronchitis and pneumonia before that. When it started clearing and I started being able to breathe for the first time, oh my God the lung surface was so expanded that I was getting air onto surfaces of the lung I hadn't gotten air onto for decades. I was fascinated. Things were different. Things were different in my body, and this was clearing out and there was great hope in it...Change was possible.

I think that a lot of what got translated as pain in the classes [what these students experienced as pain] was really overwork [working harder than was necessary]...A lot of us were still operating out of some sense that nothing really changes. And I think people just worked their butts off out of a sense of how difficult change was.

Ida was always trying to tell us it isn't – change is not difficult; it is the nature of things to change; change is possible and positive change is possible. If you wanted to get Ida activated all you had to do was say to her in a situation, "Well Dr. Rolf there's nothing you can do about that." And she'd go, "Humph! You can always do something about anything." And I think that was important. You can always do something about anything.[26]

Getting Rolfed by Dr. Rolf

As I continued to interview my teachers I was interested in finding out what it was like to be Rolfed by Ida Rolf herself, and what she was like as a teacher.

Peter

I had, a few months before, driven a car off a cliff and so my body was a mess, as you can imagine. I knew she was going to fix it. Oh, the first time she put me on a bench and started working on my back, I knew it. I thought I was going to barf…I had two broken vertebrae, but neither of us knew that. I could have figured it out – I mean, falling a hundred feet in a car! – but somehow it escaped the attention of those at the hospital. When she went to work on me I thought, "Oh my God she's going to fix it!" To me, pain was just a part of being alive. It wasn't any big deal; isn't everybody in pain? They should be if they're really participating. So, that first session was just miraculous, it was unbelievable…The change was extraordinary.[27]

Emmett

The best description I had of it was that it was like being loved. She was loving me, but not loving me as Emmett,

but as a member of my species. I felt like I was especially
blessed to be chosen; like a lab animal, an experiment or
something. But, there was great love and a sense of great
privilege, and also the feeling that you wanted to work *into*
her hands. I never got the feeling that I wanted to avoid
any of the sensations, no matter how intense or what you
might call painful they were. They never felt like I was
being injured. I always felt like I wanted to work into her
hands rather than away from them. Other than that I can't
describe it. [28]

Jan

My first experience with getting Rolfed by Dr. Rolf was
pretty rough, actually. I had asked to get treated by her
because I was having trouble with my knees. I had been
doing a lot of heavy lifting and "wheelbarrowing," and stuff
like that. I'd been injured a couple of times. She brought an
M.D., who I think was a psychiatrist, to my session...basi-
cally I was a demo....She took a photograph of me before-
hand and then gave me the treatment, which I found to be
very painful to the extent that I sort of had to "go away" to
let her do it.

After the session she spent I'll bet five minutes posing
me against the wall. "Now get your waist back, now get
your chest up, now let your shoulders go, *now now now*."
And then she ran back to the camera and took a picture
and pulled out the Polaroid and showed it to this guy as evidence that her treatment had worked.

"I can't believe this!" I was so glad to get out of that
bathhouse (because I was treated at the Esalen bathhouse),
that I swore I would never go back – I mean to myself. I
thought, *no way that isn't for me.* But about four days later,
when I was working on a project, I stretched, and the upper

part of my lungs opened on both sides with a sound like that of Velcro pulling apart. I got this huge breath and I stood there a minute. I said, "Oh my God, I've gotta go back. It worked!"[29]

Tom

When she [Dr. Rolf] touched you, you had the sense that a change was going to happen. A change you yearned for but didn't know what it was. You didn't have words for it; it was inchoate in that sense, unspoken, unknown but felt. It was like, "Yes! Oh yes! I've wanted that all my life. What is that? I don't even know what it is but I want it."[30]

Dr. Rolf as Teacher

Peter

The thing that was amazing about her is that she could [engage] a group of twelve people and be instructing each one of them at their level. It was quite extraordinary. I used to watch this, because I was doing seminars and stuff at that time too. I thought, I've never met anybody like this. She could talk as if you were the only two in the room, and everybody else would be getting it as well – and there were so many different kinds of people. There was a doctor, a couple of psychotherapists, a plumber, you know, just people from totally different backgrounds – people who had relatively little skill in terms of the body…From my point of view none of us knew shit.

She had one failing as a teacher, I thought in retrospect. It was the same failing, oddly enough, that Fritz Perls had. It involved a tendency to assume [that we had] the same level of sophistication educationally as they [Perls

"You all saw the little tree at the side of the front door," she [Ida] began. "Well that tree is known as the 'Ego Tree.' I would like you all to hang your egos on that tree as you come through the door into class each day. You may pick them up again on the way home."…I believe a seed was planted on that day and that the tree that grew from it is still bearing fruit, and I am grateful.
– PETER MELCHIOR,
REMEMBERING IDA
ROLF, 39, 41.

and Rolf] had. So she would spout these names like, "Everyone knows *blah blah blah…*" Everyone would sit there and go [he makes a blank face], like everyone was afraid to say no, and then they'd turn over and whisper to one another, "Do you know who that guy is?" A lot went by that way. Well, we didn't have that kind of education that they sometimes assumed was there. They were teaching a bunch of really unsophisticated clodhoppers to do this very sophisticated work…some of us were no more than juvenile delinquents.[31]

I never asked Emmett directly what Dr. Rolf was like as a teacher. From the rest of his interview, however, I would say that he was probably attracted by her breadth of knowledge and her ability to answer his questions and challenge him in a very deep way. I venture to guess that at times there was a meeting of two great minds; and that in Dr. Rolf, Emmett found an unexpected inner resonance with many of the ideas she was presenting. He did say, in the process of talking about Dr. Rolf as a metaphysician, that she liked to "disturb everybody's complacency and their little universe and how they thought it worked."[32]

Jan

I don't think I knew how she was as a teacher until I began to teach myself. Then, when I started looking for the models for *how do I want to teach* and *who do I want to teach like*, I began to think that Ida Rolf was actually…pretty strongly imbedded in what Peter Melchior called the school of denial, which is, "Well, that's pretty good, but it's not good enough. Someone like you may not be able to do it at the level that I can, but you can try." There was a very strong element of undercutting and lack of patience in her teaching. I don't fault her for this. I really think that a pioneer cannot afford time to coddle people. You see this kind of teaching in a frontline pioneer. So, my experience of her as a teacher was that she was absolutely determined, really relentless, seldom kind.[33]

Tom

She was scary as hell. You know me; I tend to be fairly reserved and shy and self centered in a sense of, "Well, if anything's wrong it must be my fault. If anything is not O.K. it's because I'm not O.K." and all that stuff. So, her classes were a great opportunity for me to run that one.

Some people teach with hard love, and that was Ida. I was scared to death of her. I was there [in Rolf training audit] on approval anyway. I kept after her for two years and she kept saying no [to his doing the Rolf training].

Finally, after two years and a lot of pushing, she said, "Well, I don't know. I'll tell you what. You come to class and we'll see if you work out or not."

Every time I'd get her notice she'd yell at me. I'd get up to go to the bathroom and I'd walk across the room and I'd hear her voice: "Look at that neck. You'll never be a Rolfer with a neck like that!" The way I dealt with it was to sit right next to her and pull my chair back just out of her peripheral vision. That way I could listen to everything she said and see everything from the angle she saw things and keep track of her and feel like she wasn't keeping track of me. But of course she was…it is my belief that Ida had a thing about limits. She didn't like limitations and she didn't like people living within what they perceived to be limitations when she saw that they weren't. She had a gift for seeing what was possible for people…Somebody would come in and she would start pushing to find out where their limits were; where they thought their limits were. And

Ida's capacity to see into the body was legendary …One of my last memories of Ida is sitting next to her in a class at the time when her eyesight was getting seriously bad. "Rosemary," she asked me, "who's that over there at the table on the other side of the room?" It was Joseph Heller, one of her favorite people; and I told her. "Joseph," she said, "it's under your third finger."

— ROSEMARY FEITIS, REMEMBERING IDA ROLF, 52.

once she found where she thought their limits were, she'd push harder against their resistance to show them that "you are not limited there...You are not as limited as you think you are."

I think that a lot of people's perception of her as a teacher, as a difficult teacher, was the fact that she was pushing on people to try to get them past their perceived limitations. And it came from a strong desire for people to be able to move on in every way, to evolve.[34]

She knew you, and it wasn't [just] her idea [of you] – it *was* you. It was you asking through her, I guess, somehow. I have another vision of Ida, another thing that helped me to understand. What I noticed with her was that...I started to call it the "parabolic mirror." She acted like a parabolic mirror. Whatever you threw at her came back at you multiplied. So if somebody would come in and they would be grumbling about her – you know, they would have some kind of antagonism toward her – she'd throw it right back at them, doubled, without an instant's delay. If you came at her with love, that's what you'd get back. It was the funniest thing that whatever people brought to her she just reflected it back magnified.[35]

* * *

Dr. Rolf had cast her net at Big Sur, California, and some of the first teachers of Rolfing, later to be my teachers, were captured there by the profound experience of meeting this remarkable woman. They were deeply touched by the experience of Rolfing and by Dr. Rolf, and were willing to go to great lengths in order to become trained in Rolfing.

I too had a similar experience when I was Rolfed by Ed Taylor in Tucson, Arizona, around 1976. The feeling that my body could change, and that I could experience a different way of moving and being in the world were right up there with the top-two life-changing experiences of my time on earth so far. I too went to Esalen Institute in the early-to-mid 1970s, but did not run into Dr. Rolf there. I was busy studying Gestalt therapy, the work developed by Fritz Perls; but I studied with Dick Price, one of the founders of Esalen Institute.

I did get to meet Dr. Rolf though. I had just completed my basic Rolf Practitioner training with Emmett Hutchins and Tom Wing in April of 1978. I came to Boulder for the Annual Meeting of Rolfers that is held each year. Dr. Rolf gave a presentation there; it was her last time to be present at an Annual Meeting before her death in 1979. I remember sitting in the Rolf room at the Pearl Street building in Boulder. Dr. Rolf was wheeled in her wheelchair and the whole room of Rolfers stood and applauded as she stood before the lectern to give her last talk. It was an electric moment and one I shall never forget.

Endnotes, Chapter 1

[1] Rolf, Ida P. "The Boy Logan Series." Archival video footage. Rolf Institute, undated. Probably around 1972.
[2] Guild for Structural Integration: General Information and Training Programs. Boulder, Colorado: The Guild for Structural Integration, 2001-2005, 7.
[3] Connolly, Lisa. "Ida Rolf." Human Behavior. May, 1977. Reprinted by The Rolf Institute of Structural Integration.
[4] Feitis, Rosemary. Ida Rolf Talks About Rolfing and Physical Reality. New York: Harper and Row, 1978, 3.
[5] Guild for Structural Integration, 7.
[6] Prichard, Robert. A film of a lecture by Dr. Rolf entitled "An Introduction to Structural Integration." The Rolf Institute, 1974.
[7] Rolf, Ida. "Rolfing Structural Integration: Gravity: An Unexplored Factor in the More Human Use of Human Beings." Reprinted from The Journal of the Institute for Comparative Study of History, Philosophy and the Sciences by The Rolf Institute, 1962, 3.

8 Rolf, Ida P. *Rolfing: The Vertical Experiential Side to Human Potential*. Blackwood, New Jersey, March, 1977. Reprinted by The Rolf Institute, Boulder, Colorado.
9 Ibid.
10 Melchior, Peter. Interview. Lyons, Colorado. March 4, 2004.
11 Feitis, Rosemary. Interview. New York, New York. March 26, 2004.
12 Sultan, Jan. Interview. Espanola, New Mexico. March 14, 2004.
13 Hutchins, Emmett. Interview. Kauai, Hawaii. June 9, 2004.
14 Wing, Tom. Interview. Olympia, Washington. March 25, 2004.
15 Feitis, *Ida Rolf Talks About Rolfing and Physical Reality*. 13.
16 Melchior, Interview.
17 Hutchins, Interview.
18 Ibid.
19 Ibid.
20 Sultan, Interview.
21 Wing, Interview.
22 Ibid.
23 Melchior, Interview.
24 Hutchins, Interview.
25 Sultan, Interview.
26 Wing, Interview.
27 Melchior, Interview.
28 Hutchins, Interview.
29 Sultan, Interview.
30 Wing, Interview.
31 Melchior, Interview.
32 Hutchins, Interview.
33 Sultan, Interview.

Part II
The Basics

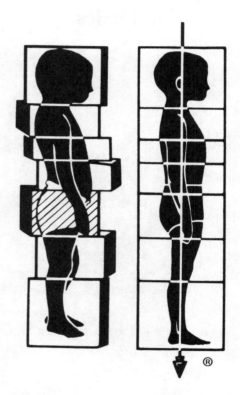

Figure 2.1 The Rolf Logo

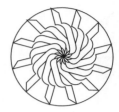

2

Basic Principles

Many people ask me, "What exactly is Rolfing? Is it like massage or chiropractic?" My initial and simplest response is to say that it is different from both of these forms because it has a unique intention and vision. My fifty-cent version of an answer is to show them the Rolf logo on my card. (*See* Figure 2.1) Looking it over they immediately point to the disorganized blocks and say, "Yes, that's me." I then go on to explain that Rolfing is a process of realigning those blocks so that one moves more toward the body shown with the blocks stacked one on top of the other.

Rolfers work in the connective tissue system of the body. This will often result in changes at the skeletal level, but we do not work directly on the bones in the way a chiropractor does, nor with the same vision and intent as a massage therapist. The most basic premise is that we are looking at relationships of the major segments of the body: head, shoulders, pelvis, and legs, and how they are organized around a vertical line of conscious intention. This assumes that the client will be a conscious participant in the process, and in the ongoing changes after initial work.

A key factor in Rolfing is the consideration of the role of gravity in the functioning of the human being, both on an immediate physical level, and on a level of ongoing evolution. There are several basic principles (like the plasticity of the body, and "the Line") that Dr. Rolf explored as she developed and taught the work, which will be presented and briefly discussed here. In later chapters they will be covered in more depth.

Plasticity of the Body

The body is flexible, a fluid energy field that is in a process of change from the moment of conception until the moment of death.

— DON JOHNSON, THE PROTEAN BODY, 2.

Plasticity is the ability of something to change shape without breaking. Connective tissue demonstrates this ability for change and responds to the warmth, pressure, and intelligence of the Rolfer's hands by stretching and changing shape somewhat the way taffy does when it is warmed up. Have you ever tried to eat cold taffy? It's a lot of work for the jaws, but when you work it a bit and warm it up, it begins to feel pliable and stretchy. The chemistry of the connective tissue of the body actually changes from a harder substance called "gel" to more of a "sol" or solution. Just as the shape of the body changes when falls, accidents and trauma happen, so it has the potential to be reshaped.

I was struck by the amazing plasticity and adaptability of the body of a client with extreme scoliosis. In scoliosis (or lateral curvature of the spine), the ribs must follow the spine, as each of the typical ribs is attached to the facet joints of two vertebrae. In an extreme scoliosis such as this man had, his ribs had to accommodate somehow for the bend in the spine and in so doing were bent almost at right angles. When I first began to lightly work with the client on his side with this convex side up, I at first thought, "What is this – it feels like the scapula, but it can't be, it's in the wrong place." Then I realized, "Wow, these are *ribs* pointing like this!"

The fascia – or connective tissue which surrounds all bones, muscles, ligaments, organs, nerves, blood vessels…every structure in the body – is considered the *organ of form*, and the matrix in which communication happens. When I feel into the tissue with the pressure of my hands, it feels like a contact improvisation. I put in information, or ask a question with my hands, and the tissue responds back with a myriad of signals, tactile feeling, and physical as well as emotional information. Because structure is a determining factor in function, then the health of the fascia is a major part of appropriate function.

Gravity as the Therapist

One way to get peoples' attention is to get them out of pain. Without the promise of some basic relief, not many would be consciously signing up for a course in personal evolution, or entertaining the possibility of moving beyond the absence of illness to the fullness of health. It is natural, therefore, for healers and teachers to go the route of "fixing" people. These are laudable and necessary skills, and many Rolfers have developed refined and creative ways to do this. Dr. Rolf herself took on people with some intense pathology.

Structural Integration carries a broad scope of ways to work. While it is a powerful tool for the relief of pain, it accomplishes this through bringing length and space into the body, and by relating the major segments of the body to each other and to the vertical, more than by working directly on pathology. "Gravity is the therapist,"[1] Dr. Rolf would say, indicating that the relief of symptoms was due more to the realignment of the body so that gravity becomes an energizing rather than a depleting force. Considering that gravity might actually help a structure toward syntropy (the tendency for a system to maintain order) rather than entropy (the tendency for a system to break down) places SI in the area of physics as well as physiology. Gravity being an energy field, and the body having its own energy field, the relationship of these

A Rolfer works with gravity; he understands the gravitational pull in everything that a human being does, 24 hours a day, 364 days a year, from the moment he gets out of his mother's womb. From that day until the day the undertaker catches up with him, gravity does not take a vacation.

– IDA P. ROLF

...when the body gets working appropriately, the force of gravity can flow through. Then spontaneously, the body heals itself.

– IDA P. ROLF

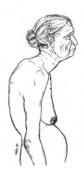

Figure 2.2
Forward head, side view
From The Endless Web *by*
R. Louis Schultz, Ph.D. and
Rosemary Feitis, D.O.
Used with permission.

fields to each other is an important factor in optimal functioning of physical structure. The force of gravity becomes an energizing force that flows harmoniously through the system.

Imagine if the weight of the head (about fifteen pounds) was positioned on the neck so as to pull the neck forward into an exaggerated secondary curve. (*See* Figure 2.2) Realize that there are countless nerves and blood vessels that go through the neck and into the medulla and rest of the brain. Think about the force of gravity exerting pressure on this placement pattern over an extended period of time. One can guess that the functions of vision and basic physiological processes would be far less than optimal. In contrast, imagine the head balanced over the cervical vertebrae, supported by a normally lifted ribcage, allowing for full breath, supported in turn by a horizontal pelvis with hips, knees, and feet in the proper relationship of support. Gravity interacting with that system will have a different effect. (*See* Figure 2.3)

Rolfing (SI) holds this broader vision of integration within the gravity field. Rolfers look for the manifestation of what is innate in the being. The genius of this work is the combination of the depth and breadth of vision, the specific knowledge of physical structure and the direct intervention into the fascial systems.

The Line

Practitioners in many types of bodywork over the years have been aware that posture (or the position of the body in space) is important to health. Yet, as children and young adults, many of us were trained in a less than optimal type of "bodywork," as we were told to "suck in your gut, shoulders back, and stand up straight." The military posture of attention, which actually tends to cut off awareness, contains this same sense of forced uprightness made with an effort of will.

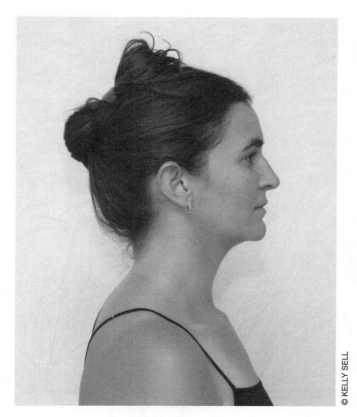

© KELLY SELL

Figure 2.3
Aligned head, side view

The line of uprightness that was Dr. Rolf's vision was to be accomplished with a natural ease and grace – a result of having given the body the length, space, and order it would need to accomplish this with little or no effort. This stance has a narrower base of support than the martial arts stance, for example, which lowers the center of gravity in readiness for attack. The narrower base gives a sense of lift, and a preparedness to move in any direction. It does not assume threat from the outside, nor make any

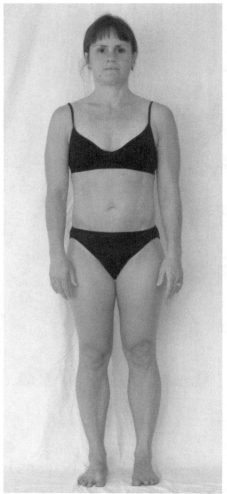

© KELLY SELL

Figure 2.4
Aligned body, front view

demands, in either a passive sense ("I need something from you")
or an aggressive sense ("I'm ready for attack"). It is simply an easy
presence: The position of the arms is neutral, neither protecting

oneself nor giving away one's power. The gaze is straightforward with a relaxed non-demanding gaze, as if the eyes originate from the back of the head. The head is level, neither down or turned in a submissive attitude, nor up in a superior or proud attitude. Everything suggests alive, neutral presence that is ready for whatever interaction is needed at the time. (*See* Figure 2.4)

An interesting study was done years ago with prisoners. Convicted muggers were shown videos of various people walking down a street and asked to pick out the people they might choose to hit on. The muggers invariably picked people whose attention was unfocused, whose structures were more random and less ordered, who were slumping or extremely rigid, and who were uncentered within themselves. Obviously the body language was clear that a person who had some structural integrity and order, as well as awareness, would not be such an easy target.

The concept of the line in Rolfing/SI is not so much postural as it is relational – that there is order around a central principle. "Man is a something built around a line,"[2] Dr. Rolf said. This statement suggests that potential for a higher order, a greater possibility for how to be in relationship to a core principle of evolving life, lies in the intention of order around a verticality that is *felt*, rather than accomplished in a finite and linear way.

Our body is a machine for living. It is organized for that, it is its nature. Let life go on in it unhindered and let it defend itself, it will do more than if you paralyze it by encumbering it with remedies.

– LEO TOLSTOY

Segmentation

The body consists of the large segments of head, shoulders, torso, pelvis, and legs. In an upright structure such as the human body, these large segments must balance over each other for order and integration to occur. This general "building blocks" outline is shown on the "little boy" Rolf logo, which was taken from actual photographs of a child with whom Dr. Rolf worked. These segments can be rotated, twisted, tilted, and pulled in many intricate ways, and where one is out of alignment, the others will all

The body is the personality exploded in three dimensions.

— IDA P. ROLF

...no situation exists in a human which a psychologist would diagnose as a feeling of insecurity or inadequacy unless it is accompanied by a physical situation which bears witness to the fact that the gravitational support is inadequate.

— IDA P. ROLF

respond to compensate. Therefore it is difficult to relieve neck problems and pain due to a forward head, for example, without looking at the underlying support system: the head rests on the cervical vertebrae, the ribs attach to the thoracic vertebrae which rest on the lumbar vertebrae, sacrum and pelvis. "De hip bone connected to de leg bone, de leg bone connected to de foot bone," as the song goes.

Many neck problems originate in the feet, legs and pelvis, and the compensatory pattern will manifest all the way up through the neck and into the cranium. A scoliosis can be felt clearly in the cranium and in the shape of the palate. Often Dr. Rolf would use homey examples like groceries in a grocery bag to describe how segments of the body had shifted within the fascial network. The idea of large body segments is a helpful and basic way to begin looking for integration in structure.

Character

The fact that character or personality manifests directly in physical structure gives the Rolfing practitioner a direct and simple way to affect old psychological patterns of behavior without trying to play psychotherapist with the client. Rather than starting with thought or emotions, and tracing their effects on the body, we can begin with the structure of the body. A person who is more integrated physically, meaning that they have freer movement, more bodily awareness, and better alignment around the vertical, seems to be more aware on the mental and emotional level, and freer in the way that he or she relates to the environment. As Rolfers, we can see that enabling the body to take a more appropriate relationship to a vertical line of motion begins to allow movement in the mental and emotional layers as well.

I also surmise that belief systems can be maintained in the fascial layers. An example of a belief system might be that "the world is a threatening and fearful place." A person with that belief system will have certain protective patterns of holding that I might be able to feel as a particular layer of hard, resistant and unconscious connective tissue. Working with these tissues I might touch on this belief as a system of holding patterns that might have been established in early childhood. Thoughts tend to revolve like a mass around a particular belief system, and if you can "catch" the core of it, then the whole constellation of thoughts can be released. The same thing happens in the body – the tissue begins to move and release when the belief system is contacted. I experience that the whole "thing" will start to move right under my hands.

With a client who carries his/her body in a defeatist attitude of dropped chest, slumped posture, forward rounded shoulders, and a feeling of not wanting to take up much space, few if any words need be said initially. Rather, that psychological pattern is directly addressed as the Rolfing works directly in the held tissues of the chest to give more lift, space, and breath.

Once a person becomes aware of a pattern, then he or she has the option to will a change. It often seems much easier to do that physically. If you slump all the time and you become aware of that behavior – actually *feeling* the effects of slumping – then you know you have the option to change that pattern. You can start to do what you want. Adjusting your posture, you begin building up this experience in the physical body, realizing that when you become aware of something, you can change it. It is encouraging for people to think that they can, at least up to a point, change physical structure and the way it is aligned. Then, they can apply the same awareness-leading-to-change process to the mind. Such application is now familiar and less frightening, because they have experienced it in the physical. These experiences are great for learning about taking responsibility.

The innermost belief for everyone I have worked with is always, "I am not good enough."
– LOUISE L. HAY, YOU CAN HEAL YOUR LIFE, 12.

Maturation

When you watch a child growing, especially in the first two to three years, you see how his or her options increase. At first there is only the option of turning the head, moving the whole arm or leg in random large muscle movements. The fingers are able to grasp something, but the function of the opposable thumb has not yet developed. Muscles are not yet clearly defined and only have gross action in broad general movements. As children begin to crawl and then to walk, slowly the muscles needed for these actions become more delineated and defined. They learn to pick things up, to have small muscle coordination in the fingers and hand that allows drawing or carefully placing small objects where they want them. The process of maturing involves being able to make choices and act on them appropriately.

As I'm sure is obvious to us all, many adults in their thirties, forties, fifties and beyond have not fully matured. Perhaps all of us have potential to continue maturing for the rest of our lives! Rolfing aids us in that process by physically separating muscle groups that have been glued together and are acting as one. "When the flexors flex, the extensors should extend,"[3] Dr. Rolf would point out. If you flex your arm at the elbow, the triceps muscle must extend in order to allow the biceps muscle to flex with the least amount of effort to accomplish the desired result. When the hip flexors and psoas contract to bring the thigh forward in walking, the hamstrings must lengthen.

When you watch little children learning to walk, you can notice how they use their feet, knees, and thighs as one unit, with the weight falling from side to side as they try to balance the torso above. You can also see this same pattern in some people as they age. In normal walking, the psoas muscle acts as an anterior support for the lumbars as it contracts. Thus, in optimal walking, movement goes through the spine.

Maturation, or having each muscle do its job and only its job, gives a look and feel of fluid grace in movement. The movement is free of history, thus giving the individual a range of options and the ability to choose what is necessary.

Time

The factor of time is important to consider in Rolfing, which is a process of deep and ongoing release of long-held patterns in the flesh, but also a process of reorganization, bringing the body to a new order around the vertical. Even in an adult, the process of maturation, or the ability to discriminate, to have more options, can be realized over time.

Growth patterns can become stunted or stopped due to trauma at a young age. One can see sometimes that the legs supporting an adult body look small and weak. A look at only the legs, then at only the upper body, may reveal that the two segments don't seem to match. The legs seem like those of a child supporting the body of an adult.

Sickness comes on horseback, but goes away on foot.
– WILLIAM C. HAZLI

When prospective clients ask how long Rolfing/Structural Integration® will take, I tell them it is a process, and often use the example of making a bed. You can't get the wrinkle out where the wrinkle is; instead, you have to go around the bed and make many moves before you can get the sheet straight. For the more mental types who ask this question, I use the example of the Rubix cube. You have to make several other moves before you can make the move that might really shift things.

As the body becomes more aligned with gravity, changes go on taking place over time. A study with children, done in 1981 by Robert Toporek, yielded some very dramatic photographs of changes in the childrens' bodies over the process of the Ten-Session Series, one year later and three years later. Significantly, there were as many if not more changes documented in those pictures

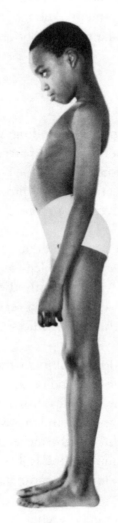 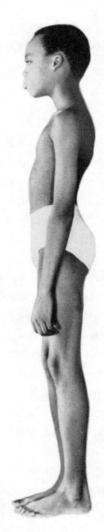

Before one session   *After ten sessions*

Figure 2.5
"J.C." in four stages
From The Promise of Rolfing Children *by Robert Toporek.*
Used with permission.

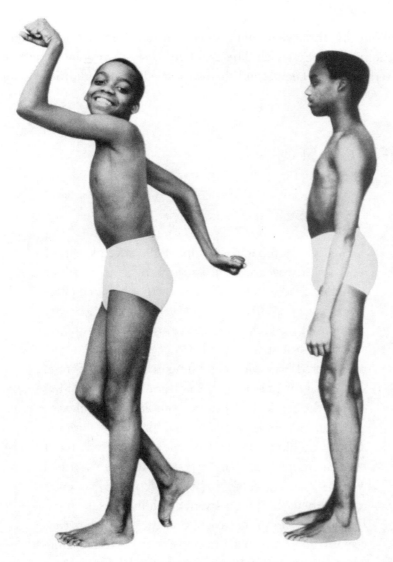

One year later, with no further Rolfing   *Three years later, with no further Rolfing*

after one and three years, without any further Rolfing, as there were in the first Ten Sessions! The children were growing *into* the new pattern that had been established with the initial work. (*See* Figure 2.5)

ERIC'S STORY

Eric is a professional musician who tours with a band both in the United States and Europe.

For years I wanted to try Rolfing. After several years of working on psychological issues through more traditional methods, I felt stuck. I knew that habitual emotional patterns were held in the body, which is why my mental insights often went nowhere. I was doing Anusara Yoga at the time I was getting Rolfed, and I was amazed how each complimented the other. Yoga was a way of practicing what I got through Rolfing during the week. I feel more confident and relaxed, stronger, less afraid of people and also more comfortable being alone. Several people have noted that I take up more space (in a good way). I've noticed women reacting more positively to me. I've even noticed new thinking patterns, valuing myself more. But, as one part of me grows, there are old habits that remain, and I see that I have work to do to continue what has started through Rolfing and bring it into every area of my life. Rolfing gave me a good reference point of feeling more confident and safe in the world, but I have to continue to choose that reality in the face of old habits that won't just lay down and die.

* * *

The tremendous potential that is available with the reordering of structure gives many options for exploration, both within us and within the body of work of Rolfing/Structural Integration. Yet, on another level, the simple power of the hands on the flesh, the feel under the hands of the aliveness, the character, the quality of the tissue, gives both the practitioner and the client a clear avenue for developing awareness. Integration, or the relationship of parts to a central whole, can be as direct as working to unwind the hardened flesh around an old ankle sprain so that the foot can relate again to the knee and hip joints, or as far reaching as how the whole pattern of reorganizing structure relates to creating a new way of relating to self and the world.

The goal of Structural Integration is the creation of order in the three dimensional body. Structural Integration is about how pieces or segments of the body are joined and how they are able to move in relation each to each...Structural Integration can change the energy body which is the man.

– IDA P. ROLF

Endnotes, Chapter 2

[1] Class notes from Rolf classes.
[2] Ibid.
[3] Ibid.

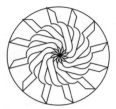

3
How Bodies Become Misaligned

It is a wonder we can function relatively normally, considering the various physical and psychological traumas most of us have endured, whether we knew it or not. The human organism is marvelously adaptable and all of our habitual patterns of structure and behavior are mechanisms we developed in order to survive. So, as we begin this exploration of the Rolfing® experience, kudos to your body/being and to mine for being here!

At the deepest level of structure is your heredity: your genes will determine whether you are tall, short, thick or thin, have certain tendencies such as flat feet, or have a generally strong or weak constitution. From there, certain tension patterns can develop in utero. Space becomes a factor as the fetus grows, especially if the mother's posture doesn't easily support the child. As Schultz and Feitis state in their book *The Endless Web*, "The child's position in the uterus is thus important in its structural development and alignment. Whether the head is to the right or to the left of the knees, where the arms are in relationship to the spine – these factors establish the individual pattern of the vertebral column. We assume that the position of the head and neck is determined by these spinal rotations. It was Ida Rolf's assumption that this relationship is established as early as the first week of pregnancy."[1]

The birth process is a major factor in influencing structure. At best, birth is somewhat stressful, significantly stressful if forceps are used or the mother is anaesthetized, or if the birth is difficult and long. The spine of a newborn has a natural C-curve with the hips tucked under. As the child begins life, he or she begins to straighten, to lift the head, to see, to explore, and to mimic adults. Thus the secondary curves of the spine develop as the child begins to crawl and later to stand and walk. Many other patterns can begin to develop in the structure in early development if, for example, the parent constantly pulls the child up by one arm, or uses especially thick diapers, or speaks sharply with an angry tone that instills the startle reflex of habitual flexion of the body. (*See* Figure 3.1) Schultz and Feitis state, "There are basically two different kinds of malfunction in the body – those caused by traumatic (external) stress and those that result from developmental (internal) stress."[2]

One of the first developmental things a newborn must learn to do is to breathe. What was the first experience of breath outside the womb like for that child? What were his or her first sights and sounds? Where was the mother, and what sense of security did her child feel? Certain restrictive breathing habits become established early, and then become limiting and eventually locked in the structure. As a Rolfer I am continually impressed that one of the first things that clients extol about their Rolfing experience is being able to breathe more freely. I am amazed that a structural deviation begun as early as birth and early childhood could be changed thirty or forty years later.

Throughout the developmental process of growth, individuals have their own timing. Trying to potty train a child before the sphincter muscles are fully developed often causes the child to

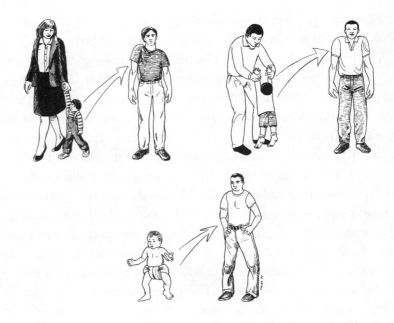

Figure 3.1
Childhood patterns affect adult posture.

tighten the whole pelvic floor in order to hold back urination or defecation. This becomes an unconscious habit in the adult.

Children mimic their parents' ways of moving, walking, and speaking. Mom and Dad are the coolest beings around, and a little child copies the behavior of the adults nearest him. When you hear your little six-year-old spouting profanities, or walking with a peculiar gait, it's great feedback about your own language and movement patterns!

Accidents and Injuries

External traumatic stress lodges in the connective tissue system of the body in the form of thickened, shortened and hardened tissue. Rotations of spine, hips, head, legs and feet form as compensatory patterns. The job of the body is to remain functional, both physiologically and psychologically. With a physiological injury such as a sprain or broken bone, the immediate reaction is swelling and hardening of the connective tissue in order to form protection from further injury. Let's say for example that Suzy, a hypothetical young woman, falls while running down a hiking trail and badly sprains her left ankle. First of all the shock of the fall dissipates through the whole fascial system in order to spread the force of the fall so it is not all received in one place. Adrenaline is released into her bloodstream; the sympathetic branch of her autonomic nervous system kicks in to mobilize the resources she will need to get herself out of danger. Luckily in this case (since I'm making this up) she was not far from the bottom of the trail and was able to hobble down to her car. After a trip to the doctor, it is determined that she did not break her ankle, but she must be on crutches for a couple of weeks. Maybe after a month or two she is able to walk again, but already carries the habit pattern of favoring the left leg. Because her body is young and strong, she heals quickly and soon is back to her full level of sports. But, a year or so later, Suzy develops a mysterious pain in her left hip that she notices when running. Being an intelligent girl, she decides to try some Rolfing. The Rolfer notices that Suzy walks on the outside of her left foot and the tissue around the peroneal muscles on the lateral side of her lower leg is holding her ankle in a position that does not allow for full flexion of the joint in the proper plane. As the rest of the body is stacked upon the ankles and feet, the Rolfer sees many compensations running through Suzy's legs, hips and up into her spine and neck from the adjustments her body had to make in order to balance. The shock of her original fall, that was dissipated through her fascial system, is now lodged there as a pattern of compensation. A Rolfer could work on her hip alone, where she is feeling the pain, but the real problem could lie in the

Not everything that is faced can be changed; but nothing can be changed until it is faced.
— JAMES BALDWIN

What we intend to do with ourselves literally shapes us: how we choose to deal with our environment, our fears and other emotions; the types of activity we choose; the lifestyle we create; the food we eat; our programs of exercise and stress reduction.
– DON JOHNSON, *THE PROTEAN BODY*, 11.

misalignment of her ankle. The Rolfer will work to follow and release all of the places where the fascia is shortened and stuck from that original fall. This simple example demonstrates how an injury can cause pain and malfunction in areas of the body other than where the original trauma happened.

In all types of accidents that befall people, the body deals brilliantly, compensating for such traumas. Whiplash from car accidents, another common yet insidious injury, often shows up as back and neck pain months after the event. Whiplash has a particular "feel" to it that I have learned to recognize – as though layers of tissue have been yanked into disorganized relationships and then frozen there, like hard dry leather. As the more surface holding begins to release, I begin to feel the most intricate and complicated arrangements of tissue around the original injury.

The different accidents people have had are innumerable, and some of these traumas are buried so deeply in the tissue that a person doesn't even remember having been hurt. In my intake interview I always ask my clients whether they have had any accidents, injuries or trauma of any kind. Over and over again I find that once we get working all kinds of things come forth from the body's own cellular memory. One client of mine had chronic sciatic pain. We worked and worked, and he got free of most of it, but there was this remaining "strange look" in the structure of his upper back and right shoulder that I could somehow never get a handle on. After working together off and on for about two years, he finally remembered that he had been run over by a truck when he was a little kid. The ground had been soft and the truck tire had run over his right shoulder and just missed his head! Once he had that memory and we worked some more on the shoulder, his back pain went away.

When a person undergoes surgery there is a change of structure that must then be integrated into the rest of the body. If a tumor is removed from the abdominal area, or the gall bladder or piece of the colon is removed, the body must somehow reorganize around that space. All the layers of muscle that were cut through must heal and knit together. Often, abdominal surgery causes a shortening all through the layers of abdominal muscles, as adhesions form when the muscles knit together. I have often worked with people who have healed well from abdominal surgery, but they say they feel stooped over and can't stand up straight. A gentle stretching of the abdominal muscles with a bit of focus on the more obvious adhesions in the tissue can bring immediate relief.

Psychological Trauma

Sexual, physical, and psychological abuse have as much if not more far-reaching negative effects on structure and behavior than accidents do. When these things happen to a child most often the breath is affected, as shutting off breathing shuts off feelings. Common protective and survival patterns involve dissociation from the body and a sympathetic nervous-system dominance that results in an ongoing feeling of tension and anxiety. (See more on this in Chapter 11, *Trauma*.) Children (or adults) make certain decisions about themselves and about life that are reflected in their body structure and connective tissue. When breath is diminished, life itself is diminished. When the systems of the body receive less oxygen, body function is less optimal. The effects of psychological trauma may be seen in the chest that is flat and hard, or collapsed, or puffed up with the abdominal muscles pushed outward to block feeling. Sometimes the whole look of the person is one of defeat, or of just not being present to interact. Each person will have his or her own way of dealing with such trauma, yet the behavior will always be reflected in structure.

Even just the normal "slings and arrows of outrageous fortune" of life lived on Planet Earth cause changes in structure. A simple fever or illness that lays you up in bed for a few days will manifest

RANDY'S STORY

"Randy" came to Rolfing with low back pain, a general lack of energy, and too much weight for his frame. At his job he spent a lot of time on the computer, sitting with his lower back rounded, his chest dropped and his head forward. This put strain on his low back and neck, but because of the tightness in his structure he did not feel comfortable sitting more erect. Slowly, over the course of the Rolfing, his body became more open and balanced. I showed him a less stressful sitting position and encouraged him to change position more often when working at the computer and to adjust his chair and desk height to accommodate these changes. As his body became more alive during the Rolfing, Randy felt more like moving. Exercise became more enjoyable. In the end it was Randy who chose to change those habits. As he continued to come for advanced Rolfing and regular "tune ups" to keep his body open, he moved to a higher level of integration. — Betsy Sise

in structure as a drop in the rib angles and a slight increase in flexion throughout the body. Usually after a day or two of being up and about, and after maybe doing some stretching or yoga, you return to your own "normal." Yet, what then becomes the kinesthetic sense of "normal" may actually entail less range of movement than you had before the illness.

Giving birth, nursing an infant, playing sports, engaging in hobbies, working at your job, all make certain demands on the body. Even the food we feed ourselves in the form of impressions, as well as the food we eat, have effects in the fascia of the body.

No one is perfect, nor are we aiming for any static state of perfection. When body and mind are open, resilient and grounded we are better able to adapt in all situations of life, whether they are positive or negative.

Endnotes, Chapter 3

[1] Schultz, R. Louis, Ph.D. and Rosemary Feitis, D.O. *The Endless Web: Fascial Anatomy and Physical Reality.* Berkeley, California: North Atlantic Books, 1996, 15.
[2] Ibid., 21.

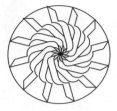

4
The Rolf Line

One of the most important and unique principles of Rolfing is the concept of organizing the body around a vertical line that is felt as a sense of lift through the physical body. Rolfers call this "the Rolf Line" (or simply, "the Line"), and it is one of the major concepts that sets Rolfing apart from other forms of bodywork, although many Rolfing techniques have spread throughout the bodywork community.

Rolfing also includes a particular vision about human structure and what might be most optimal balance for an upright being. It considers fields: the field of gravity, the electromagnetic field of the body as a whole, as well as the myriad of fields created by individual organs such as the heart. Dr. Rolf's genius was to reach beyond what science was telling her at the time to intuit that "man was a something built around a line,"[1] and that man lives in an environmental field, the gravitational field, with which he constantly interacts from conception to death.

Ida Rolf envisioned and experienced this Line as beginning at the bottoms of the feet and going up and out through the top of the head. This Line is not located in a specific structural space, but is an experience of lift. (Figures 4.1 and 4.2 show two people with quite different structures, each of whom give a good, basic demonstration of the Line.) When I tune into my body in a standing posture I can feel the Line from just in front of my heels, up the core of my legs, along the line of the psoas and up the front of my spine to the palate and out the top of my head. Immediately after a good Rolfing session, especially, I can let go of holding myself up in space and feel a support coming up through my body that gives me a feeling that my body is just standing upright without much effort from me.

The word "line" implies a static and immovable aspect, but in my experience the Rolf Line is alive with movement and energy, a dynamic experience of the peace of grounded verticality. Dr. Rolf put it well when she said:

> This is what Rolfers are doing: we are lifting a body up...It all sounds so much alike: I will lift up my head; I am lifting toward the Lord; I am lifting toward the mountain. All religious thinking has tended to understand that there was a lifting up in terms of growth in the spiritual realm.[2]

This concept of the Line is what links the integration of structure in the realm of physics and physiology to the realm of metaphysics, and is the bridge between physical reality and non-physical reality. Dr. Rolf was exploring the possibility of a person who was integrated in the gravitational field being grounded through the earth with the feet, with the head lifted and open to the cosmos, and yet able to function in the world – the relationship between horizontal and vertical. How does one aspire vertically while still being able to relate horizontally to the world? Perhaps a symbol for this could be the cross – the mysticism of the right angle. In a purely physical sense, when fascia around the joints

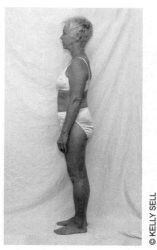

© KELLY SELL

Figure 4.1
A good "Line," side view

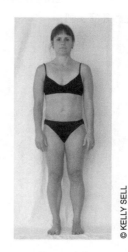

© KELLY SELL

Figure 4.2
A good "Line," front view

begins to act in a horizontal manner, the support for vertical experience naturally emerges.[3]

The Line is something that must be transmitted and taught. Dr. Rolf used to say that we were more educators than therapists. As a Rolfer, I must teach the client ways to learn how to become more conscious in his or her everyday movement habits and remember often to "find" (just become conscious of) the bottoms of the feet, the top of the head, and feel the connection all the way through. This is not easy, and most folks will probably not focus on the Line, or on Rolfing as a growth path. Yet even so, growth takes place unconsciously. I can see it in my clients, particularly ones with whom I have worked for a number of years. I watch them begin to make decisions that are more "in line" with who they really are.

Emmett Hutchins once told me that if I could find the space between the two sides of my body I would know who I am. I have found what I call "the space in front of the spine" and it is alive with lift, ease, openness and wisdom. Have I found out who I am? I would say that now and then I get a glimpse when that space called "the Line" is especially clear and bright. I also know that whenever I feel really funky emotionally, I also feel off in my body – short and constricted. Finding where "up" is, and taking my attention back to the front of the spine, I can sometimes watch the turmoil on the surface from a deeper place. (Believe me, by no means always!)

Each Rolfer and Rolfee will have a different feeling about this Line. It is a personal experience as much as a theory or concept, and involves the intention and conscious will of the client as well as of the Rolfer. In our classes with Emmett Hutchins, he often challenged us to meditate on this Line in a standing posture. According to my class notes he described the Line as "imaginary, as it has no density and molecules. It's like a cosmic smile of space and radiation. You have to intend it and believe in it before it becomes real."[4] Peter described the Line as "a vector of gravitational response."[5] Ida Rolf described the Line as "a continuous now."[6] Janie French and Annie Duggan described it as follows: "The Line is a space of knowing around which we organize and respond."[7]

PAMELA'S STORY

Pamela, a client of mine in Vermont, had a severe scoliosis — severe enough that her doctor wanted to do surgery to place rods in her back. Pamela of course was hesitant, as this major surgery can have varying results. After giving her the Basic Ten Series, I continued to Rolf her extensively during my time in Vermont. With the Rolfing and a lot of focused work on her part with specific exercise, she was able to stay active and relatively pain free over the eight years that I knew her. We set up a maintenance program of Rolfing once a month and were thus able to stay one jump ahead of further deterioration in the degree of her spinal curve. Pamela had more freedom of movement and more rib excursion during breathing than some of my clients with far less severe problems. Although Pamela's spine was curved, it moved and she was able to find a conscious center line through her body. — Betsy Sise

The material universe is bound together as though it were one, and its various parts are as interdependent as our own vital functions, none of which can be affected without influencing the whole body. Therefore, humans aren't citizens merely of this world, but of the universe in all its parts, visible and invisible.
– ROBERT C. FULFORD, D.O., DR. FULFORD'S TOUCH OF LIFE, 21.

The concept of the Line makes us realize that health is far more than just the absence of illness. There are levels of health and wholeness that most of us have not yet experienced. How many of us live in joyfulness with ease and grace of movement, and strength and power that is flexible? How many of us feel a relaxed letting go into a sense of vertical lift? Since we live our human lives in a gravitational field we often forget that the relationship of that field with our own energy field is vital to our health and well being. Whatever keeps us from experiencing alignment with vertical in the physical body, and with resting in Truth on the greater level, is ultimately the beginning of disease, or lack of appropriate relationship to the nature of what is.

Relaxation and letting go, though key factors in both physical health and spiritual growth, demand a certain discrimination and awareness. In a physical sense, to relax without an appropriate relationship to gravity means that the body has no inner support on which to rest, and thus it tends to support itself with the extremes of collapse and rigidity. If this metaphor is carried to the spiritual and emotional levels, again, without proper alignment to spiritual values and principles, one risks letting go into a circular indulgence of emotions, or a relaxing into ego desires that actually can keep one blocked. There must be an appropriate and aware relationship to verticality, both spiritually and physically.

Verticality, space, relationship, integration, discrimination, movement, flow – these words describe a person integrated in relation to a principle of uprightness, able to discriminate between appropriate and inappropriate behavior within their surroundings, and able to allow spaciousness in mind and body in which to move.

I love it when certain truths show up in different contexts. Reading the above paragraph, I am reminded of a dance teacher I once had in Tucson – Barbara Mettler of the Tucson Creative Dance Center. She had a gorgeous circular dance studio that was designed by Frank Lloyd Wright, and she had a unique way of teaching in this beautiful ritual space. According to Barbara, first you get the instrument (the body) to be free in its expression in a great variety of ways as it deals with space, time, shape and form. Then you begin developing awareness of your body as you move in relationship to other bodies in the space. Finally, when your freedom of movement and awareness has developed, you begin to use control, so that you remain in constant balance between allowing yourself to be moved by the creative force, and initiating the movement that the dance needs to have happen. The Rolf Line contains the essence of that same balance with freedom, awareness and control. There is some use of will to lift the top of the head, but there is, at the same time, an opening for the creative force of gravity to move through the system so there is neither collapse nor striving, but a conscious allowing.

The Teachers Speak about the Rolf Line

Emmett Hutchins

Well, Ida had several definitions for Structural Integration, but one of them was to create a standing polarity between the top of the head and the bottom of the feet – to have one Line that goes from the top of your head and ends up at the ankles. You don't see this in very many members of our species. At best I think people have to look at that as an ideal. But the Line is the principle around which all of Ida's physics and metaphysics are built.

She called the Line transcendental, meaning that [it included] not only all the Newtonian physics, not only the physics of the blocks, stresses and strains, the balance and the fulcrums, and all the mechanical (or even non-mechanical) aspects of structure [and] that they're all relationship aspects of structure. So they all have to do with Newtonian physics and can be explained in terms of balance, and that all [that] has to do with balance around a line. There is no other way that way human beings are balanced. Also, all of her [Dr. Rolf's] metaphysics is around the idea of the Line. The Line put human structures in

All living bodies are energy systems, which strive to maintain themselves in a state of dynamic equilibrium.
– ROBERT C. FULFORD, D.O., DR. FULFORD'S TOUCH OF LIFE, 187.

agreement with the field in which they lived…It's what made individual human beings join the universe as a whole. You do it through the Line because that is the thing that holds the earth together. That's what makes trees grow straight up and down and makes buildings stand up. And when you get a true Line in your body you become weightless, just as a house does not feel weight.

The *theory* says that you are going to feel weightless. I don't know that; I've not gotten complete weightlessness in normal consciousness. But, very clearly I feel much more weightless than I ever have in my life. Every year I get lighter and that doesn't mean that I lose weight. It has very little to do with my pounds. It's just the basic fact that Mother Earth cannot lift me up in the air any harder than I am willing to give weight to her.[8]

Peter Melchior

[The Line] was the metaphysic upon which the whole thing [Rolfing] was based. It was the idea that a different relationship between a person and the earth was possible, and that the way to that was organization around a Line, and that that Line was the transmission. She used to say [that the Line went] from the center of the earth to a far star…you know I got the feeling that to her we were events on a line. We were like a little something – a bead on this very long [curved] line – that if you carried it out indeed would circle around. It was so big that it was essentially a straight line. That's the way I got it…sometimes she was talking classical metaphysics, sometimes she was talking physics. When it came down to working on the body she wouldn't hear any metaphysics. She wanted the physical laws…

I've been doing this work for thirty-five years and I have some clients who have followed me all the way through that process. What I've seen is that a Ten-Session Series, if it is successful, succeeds in establishing a place for that Line, a "something" to work with, and that's it. If that's not done, forget about all the rest. You'll get some very nice "massagistic" kind of results, or osteopathic, or God knows what all, but you don't get Structural Integration. Unless the practitioner and the client start out [where] the main event is – establishing this Line in those first Ten Sessions – they aren't going to get it. It takes real effort, what Gurdjieff used to call "real effort." [A superior effort required to move beyond the normal mechanical responses of "sleeping" human beings, into a new realm of evolution.] I didn't understand that at first...I think it is the major responsibility [of the Rolfer] to train or to teach [or] to somehow open that idea to the client, otherwise it won't happen.

Once you had this hook up, this mysterious Line connecting you to the rest of the cosmos...your education proceeded apace. I think everybody I know who I would consider to be aware of their process (and I don't know how to even say that; there are some people who don't even care, you know, you just have a good time and do whatever you do), for anybody who's really concerned about "What the hell am I doing here?" and all that stuff, that once that hookup [to the Line] was made, life began to accelerate in some extraordinary, sometimes really uncomfortable ways. There were many things that happened historically [in Rolf classes] that lent themselves to that interpretation. In the first advanced class, nobody stayed with their [life partner]. No one ended up with [his or her wife, husband, or lover] out of that class, and Ida was very upset about

The body is a map of the universe, so you're trying to open up the body to be flexible enough to give you information about who you are – to make the instrument available...Rolfing creates a flexibility whereby things can balance around that Line, and then I can vibrate and move to express what I'm supposed to express, independent of some syndrome that I might be caught in that might be karmic or physical.

– PAUL OERTEL, DANCER

that. She called me in and said, "This is not working. It's not supposed to work this way. You are supposed to be more highly integrated."[9]

Jan Sultan

The Line is gravity. The Line *is* gravity. It's how you vision gravity's impact on the structure as a whole. As soon as you postulate the Line you've also postulated horizontals because one doesn't exist without the other. So you have a three-dimensional grid; up, down, side, side, front, back, defined by line vertically, and the horizontals that cross that – that are demanded by the vertical. So that's really the bottomline of it. I think the Line is fundamental to how you understand spatial geometry...I'm not Rolfing if I don't have gravity in there.[10]

* * *

Emmett Hutchins beautifully summed up this consideration of the Line in a paper he wrote in 1989:

Unfortunately, organization of the structure, alone, does not permanently establish this ideal super-balanced state. While fascial order may effect miracles in the relief of chronic symptoms and pain, and may commonly produce increased vitality and a new sense of general well being, it does not fully integrate a living, moving structure within the surrounding gravity field. Something is missing. The conscious will of the being that lives within the structure must be actively involved. Here we glimpse Dr. Rolf's true genius with her invention of the concept of the Line...The Line is transcendental. It forms a bridge between physical reality and the realm of pure energy, the non-physical. The Line integrates the physical structure with the gravity field. The Line joins Rolf physics and metaphysics into one clear concept. The awakening of the Line is the central challenge of her teaching. The awakening of the Line is the Rolf path for self-growth. The Line becomes our personal guide, our monitor of personal evolution. And inculcation of the Line into the very essence of our consciousness becomes our preoccupation. Dr. Rolf's vision of unlimited human potential is inseparable from this personal path.[11]

Endnotes, Chapter 4

[1] Rolf class notes.
[2] Feitis, Rosemary. Editor. *Ida Rolf Talks About Rolfing and Physical Reality*. New York, N.Y.: Harper and Row, 1978, 108.
[3] Hutchins, Emmett. Rolf class notes.
[4] Rolf class notes.
[5] Ibid.
[6] Ibid.
[7] Duggan, Annie and French, Janie. *Rolfing Movement Integration*. Unpublished paper. No date.
[8] Hutchins, Emmett. Interview. Kauai, Hawaii. June 9, 2004.
[9] Melchior, Peter. Interview. Lyons, Colorado. March 4, 2004.
[10] Sultan, Jan. Interview. Espanola, New Mexico. March 14, 2004.
[11] Hutchins, Emmett. *Structural Integration: A Path of Personal Growth and Development*. An unpublished paper written for the Guild for Structural Integration in September of 1989. Used with permission of the author.

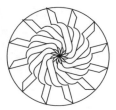

5
The Basic Ten-Session Series of Rolfing

One of the first things one hears about in Rolfing is that there is a series of sessions – some kind of progression. To begin simply, when you look at a body as a set of blocks stacked on top of each other, the bottom blocks must support the top blocks. When some of these blocks are twisted, rotated and compressed together, length and space must first be established to make room for those twisted segments to become aligned and to be able to efficiently relate to each other.

The challenges for Dr. Rolf were to establish a way for one to constantly shift one's seeing from general to specific, and to pre-pare the body for deeper changes by first creating length and space at the more superficial levels. For healers, it is always tempting to work first on the most obvious aberration, or the place where the client feels the pain. Yet, Dr. Rolf held to the principle that the alignment in the gravitational field was the reason pathology was eased in the structure, not because such pathology was worked on directly with the specific goal of palliation. Her deep and abiding interest was in the relationship between the energy field of the human and the gravitational field.

All the goals of Rolfing ultimately have to do with movement and how a person relates to the field in which she/he lives. In actuality, everything is in motion – from cells to bones to organs to a human to the planets and stars, as Nobel Prize winner Ludwig Von Bertalanffy noted in his book, *The Problems of Life*:

> This separation between a pre-established structure and processes occurring in that structure does not apply to living organisms. For the organism is the expression of an everlasting orderly process…what is described in morphology as organic forms and structures is in reality a momentary cross section through a spatio-temporal pattern. What are called structures are slow patterns of long duration, functions are quick processes of short duration.[1]

The Ten-Session Series was Dr. Rolf's way to give her students a tool for learning something that could not be taught in the abstract, but had to be experienced. She carefully developed the series with a set of goals for each session, which when followed would usually bring clearly observable results. In this way students could safely take clients through a progressive and balanced set of changes while keeping them integrated and grounded in their experience. This series was followed as a practice, a discipline, and a ritual somewhat like meditation. That is, you *just do it*…on and on…and soon you begin to learn how structure can change and come into order around a vertical line. You learn to see the whole, the parts, and how they relate. You learn to see the brilliant and intricate structural logic contained in this series of sessions. Eventually, you embody this knowledge in your own being, and then the knowledge of the Ten Series is a part of you and you can work freely with that background of vision as your safety net.

This basic Ten-Session Series later became known among Rolfers as "The Recipe." Many variations of the Recipe have been

written up and scattered around throughout the Rolfing community (and probably beyond) over the years. Originally, these copies
were not to be shared outside of the Rolf community for fear that
an untrained person could take a written recipe, use it improperly
and superficially, and call it "Rolfing." (This has in all likelihood
been done.)

No one should attempt Rolfing based on anything said in this
book without becoming fully trained as a practitioner of Rolfing -
Structural Integration. Harm can definitely be done by attempting
to try certain "moves" without understanding the whole. Rolfers
go through an extensive training of experiential, didactic and
hands-on work.

The Recipe is not a form that is laid on everyone, regardless of
their problem, although some could use it that way. Rather, the
series is meant to be used in a highly creative way that considers
each client's unique problems and personality.

Dr. Rolf would ask her students to practice this Ten Series –
and *only* the Rolfing modality – for at least five years before studying any other healing art. She saw Rolfing as a lifetime art as well
as a way of life. Teachers such as Ida Rolf and Mary Burmeister of
Jin Shin Jyutsu® spent their lives immersed in the development of
their own work. They often had other interests that related to
their work, but they exclusively practiced their own art. Mary
Burmeister once said that she practiced Jin Shin Jyutsu on herself
for eight years before she ever touched anyone else!

My Experience with the Basic Ten Series

Over the years of my own Rolfing practice I have used the
Ten-Session Series as a general framework in which to be in rela-
tionship with my client. For me, the magic is the form behind the
Ten Series not the Ten Series itself. The series provides a context

that contains great wisdom; a container in which I can explore and learn and give to the client all that I am.

I use the Ten-Session Series somewhat as I use my Rolf studio (which I call my "magic box"). My studio is a ritual space, a chamber that I have set up in which the client and I will journey together during the Ten Sessions. This careful setting up of particular boundaries allows me a certain safety within which I have great freedom. My clients know from the outset that we will work together for ten sessions, that I will be present for them all along the way as they move through their changes and experience their growth and expansion.

Even after twenty-seven years of Rolfing I still like to use this ritual journey of ten hours for the person just beginning Rolfing. It is my particular joy and interest to take someone through a process of change toward a higher order of being.

* * *

Eat right, exercise regularly, die anyway.
    – AUTHOR UNKNOWN

I hope you will come to feel from reading this chapter and the teachers' comments on this Ten-Session Series that there is far more to it than meets the eye. I feel that this Series, along with the principle of the "Line," is the core of Rolfing. It is what makes Rolfing stand out from other types of bodywork. In my experience there is no way to transmit the knowledge contained in the basic Ten Series without first embodying it in oneself and then practicing it with clients for years. This chapter, therefore, will present a "feel" for the journey and the basic progression of this Ten-Session Series, yet purposefully remain vague about specifics of the sessions.

Basic Premises of the Series

What follows is a brief review of some of the basic premises contained within this particular approach to organizing structure.

Even though it appears that the same kind of work is done on each person no matter what the problem, it is the *goals* of the sessions that provide a progressive and highly functional way to work. How these goals are achieved may be quite varied in each individual. The real art of the work is in the interaction between Rolfer and client, the communication of touch, word, and presence, the acceptance of the client where he or she is, and the transmitting of excitement and discovery – the drawing out of the client's true being.

A General Template for Balanced and Integrated Structure

When looking for a balanced structure Rolfers observe certain visual and kinesthetic key points. It is difficult to describe in linear terms something that is living in dynamic relationship with the environment without that description sounding like a model of perfection. This is definitely not the purpose of Rolfing. The following lists are attempts to give a general framework of some things we might be observing in structure when the person is standing in a neutral position. The accompanying photographs are of two women with quite different body types. Each of these women has been Rolfed and each is functioning well in her life. You can see that each demonstrates the general outline of a balanced structure, yet each has her own specific areas of challenge or "growing edge."

When looking from a side view (See Figure 5.1)
- The heels reach back giving support to the sacrum and occiput.
- Weight goes down the front of the shins; hip and knee are aligned over the ankle. The pelvis is horizontal, and the secondary curves of the spine are balanced, neither too flat, nor too exaggerated.

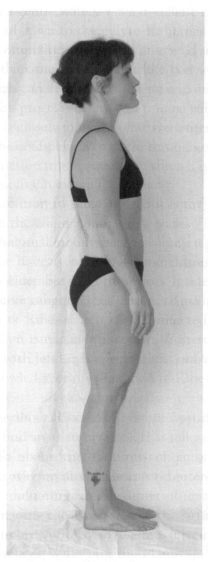

Figure 5.1
Side view

- The ribs are lifted in order to support the yoke of the shoulder girdle, and the flesh of the torso is balanced front to back, with the arm lying along the midline.
- The shoulder joint is directly over the hip joint, and there is balance between the clavicles and scapula.
- The head rests directly on top of the neck, with the eyes looking straight out.
- The ear is aligned over the shoulder.
- There is as much head in back of the atlanto-occipital joint as in front.

When looking from the front (See Figure 5.2)
- The feet are pointing straight ahead.
- There is slight lift to the lateral arch giving support to the medial arch of the foot.
- When walking, the transverse arch is used evenly, and the knees track straight ahead, indicating use of the psoas to support the lumbar vertebrae.
- The line through the psoas to the adductors is open and long enough to allow for a horizontal pelvis that is balanced right to left.
- Weight passes through the hip fascia near the hip joint, rather than being carried out along the area of the greater trochanter of the femur.
- The arms hang along the side of the body in a neutral position, neither in a protective, nor submissive posture.
- The shoulder girdle rests evenly on the ribs.
- The head is neither tilted up, down, or sideways, the sphenoid bone is balanced and the eyes look directly to the front.

When looking from the back (See Figure 5.3)
- The heels are even, directly giving support to the sacrum and occiput.

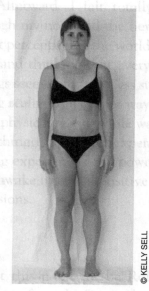

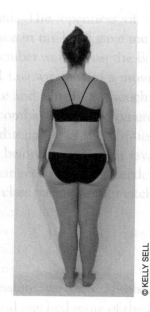

© KELLY SELL

© KELLY SELL

Figure 5.2
Front view

Figure 5.3
Back view

- When the person bends the knees, there is enough length through the gastrocnemius and soleus muscles for the Achilles tendon to lengthen, and allowing the heels to remain straight ahead without being pulled either medially or laterally.
- There is movement at the sacroiliac joints and balance between the right and left outward rotators of the hip.
- The hamstrings lengthen evenly when the knees are bent.
- The scapulas rest down on the ribs when the arms are raised to the front.
- The shoulders are even, indicating that the ribs and spine on which they rest are not rotated or dropped.
- When the hair is out of the way, you can see both ears equally and the trapezius muscle looks even, right to left.

While holding these general goals in mind, it is important to note that each person is unique, and will be unique in the way that he or she relates to gravity after Rolfing. I remember Rolfing a woman at an advanced Rolfing workshop in Scottsdale, Arizona. This woman had received a lot of good Rolfing and she also had a pronounced scoliosis. When I was working with her, she had a marvelous kinesthetic sense and awareness in her body. When she stood up after the session I was suddenly aware that I could see her clear consciousness of a vertical line of lift that went right through the middle of her curved spine. For her, in her body at that time, she was aligned around a central core of lift.

Many times the results of accidents and injuries in the connective tissue are greatly altered and relieved, but not totally eliminated. Such injuries sometimes remain as a part of the being, and are integrated into a new reality in the body/mind. History is not always totally erased, but it is changed and brought into present time in such a way that it is integrated into the rest of the structure as the person moves along his or her evolutionary path. There is no single ideal form toward which we push each person, only his or her own particular ideal form.

The most important results of an integrated structure are how the person feels about herself, her image of her body, and how she is functioning and expressing who she is in the everyday world. An ideal static posture is not the goal of Rolfing. Verticality in the gravitational field is a neutral position from which arises an alive, expressive interaction with the environment. A person becomes more human and spontaneous with less mechanistic repetition of old habit patterns.

It's not what we do that makes us Rolfers, it's what we are.
– IDA P. ROLF

Creating Space, Establishing Layers – the First Three Sessions

The first thought in looking at the structure with the stacked blocks model would be to begin at the feet as the base of support. This was the way Dr. Rolf first began, but she discovered through a foot reflexologist that work on the feet stirs up reflexes and puts stress on elimination as well as on the upper body.[2] She also noticed that if the breath wasn't open, the tissue did not change as easily or quickly.

In the first steps of this series the Rolfer establishes contact with the client, notices the client's key issue or holding pattern, and decides how to begin to create some space and resilience in the structure and how to get some energy moving through opening the breath. As the client begins to expand his breathing, the tissues become more oxygenated and thus riper for change.

As practitioners, we aim for a lift in the thorax off the pelvis in order to set up space for future changes in the pelvis. How the femur relates to the pelvis is one of the keys to bringing the pelvis to a horizontal position. The goal is to allow for an open, unrestricted pattern of breathing, length in the front of the torso, the ability for the thigh to move freely from the pelvis, and a lift of the torso off the pelvis. When the flexors flex, the extensors should extend; thus, when the thigh flexes, the hamstrings should lengthen. We begin fairly generally, working with larger, more superficial, planes of fascia, while preparing for more specific and deeper work later.

The back work in the earlier sessions begins to develop in the client an even C-curve before trying to work with unwinding rotations, or easing exaggerated secondary spinal curves. The pelvic lift is done at the end of each session to integrate changes through the body, easing length into the lumbar fascia, and allowing the 5th

Support is a relationship, not something solid.
                – IDA P. ROLF

lumbar vertebra to drop back toward the bed when the client is lying on his back.

Working with the Feet

Upon the feet rest the entire weight and balance of the body. Many problems in the back and neck originate from aberrations and misalignment in the feet and ankles.

The foot is a finely crafted balance of small bones that create three arches. The lateral arch consists of the calcaneus, cuboid, and 4th and 5th metatarsal bones. The medial arch partially rests on the lateral arch and is made up of the talus, navicular, and cuneiform bones. The metatarsal arch spans the foot horizontally

The gospel according to osteopaths is to try to go to the center to get to the cause and change it. The gospel according to Rolf is that you can't get to the center to change it until you work with the outside. The body is like an onion. To get to the center without injury you must peel it layer by layer.

– IDA P. ROLF

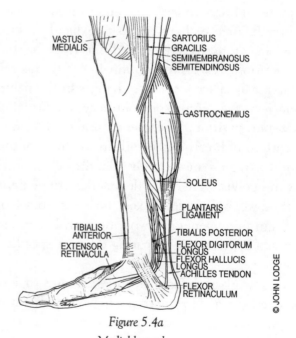

Figure 5.4a
Medial lower leg
From Rolfing: The Integration of Human Structures, *by Ida P. Rolf.*
Used with permission.

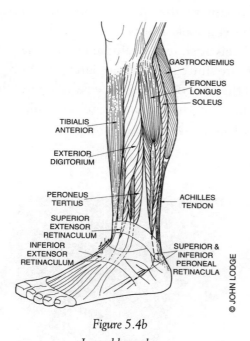

GASTROCNEMIUS

PERONEUS
LONGUS

SOLEUS

TIBIALIS
ANTERIOR

EXTERIOR
DIGITORIUM

PERONEUS
TERTIUS

ACHILLES
TENDON

SUPERIOR
EXTENSOR
RETINACULUM

INFERIOR
EXTENSOR
RETINACULUM

SUPERIOR &
INFERIOR
PERONEAL
RETINACULA

© JOHN LODGE

Figure 5.4b
Lateral lower leg
From Rolfing: The Integration of Human Structures, *by Ida P. Rolf.*
Used with permission.

at the distal joints of the metatarsal bones. By freeing the hard-ened retinaculum around the ankle and shin, the position of the foot can be changed. The tendons of the tibialis anterior and pos-terior, the flexor digitorum longus, and the flexor hallucis longus cross under the medial malleolus. (*See* Figures 5.4 a and b) The peroneus longus and brevis cross behind the lateral malleolus. These tendons form a stirrup that attaches to the plantar fascia. When the muscles of the shin and lower leg are wrenched out of balance by accident or habit pattern, the arches are affected. The feet begin to toe-out or -in, and then the tissue becomes hard and unresilient, trapping the feet in the pattern of the injury.

The placement of the heel is a key to the support of the sacrum. When you look at a person from the back, you can see whether the heels are directly centered under the ischial tuberosities, or if they are shifted medially or laterally. Work in the area of the shins and the back of the leg, especially behind the head of the fibula, will allow for changes in the relationship of the arches of the foot. (*See* Figure 5.5)

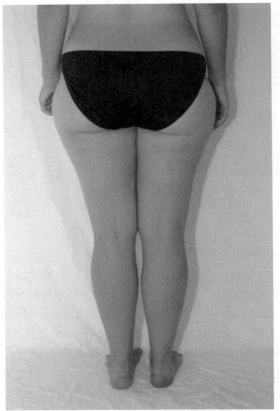

© KELLY SELL

Figure 5.5
Heels aligned under sit bones and sacrum

Layers

The early sessions of Rolfing deal directly with this concept of layers in the body. Outer compensatory layers must be eased and lengthened before deeper holding can be reached. As the client begins to breathe more freely and gain some grounding through the feet we can begin to look at the area around the 12th rib and crest of the ilium, beginning to establish a midline in the side plane of the body, as if there is a line from the head of the humerus of the shoulder down through the greater trochanter of the femur. We can begin work with the relationship of the shoulder girdle to the thorax, and the pelvis to the thorax. We can see clearly whether the shoulder girdle is rolled forward, for example, or whether the pelvis is tilted forward, and what kind of space there is around the 12th rib and quadratus lumborum. (*See* Figure 5.6, which is a drawing in movement and shows the general area of work.)

The ribs should move a bit like Venetian blinds, turning on the vertebrae as they move upward on inspiration. One should see the pelvis respond to the movement of the breath. We are looking for the shoulder girdle and pelvic girdle to move freely and separately from the thorax, yet to be related to each other.

How does one accomplish such goals with only the use of the hands? There is no way one can read about it or even write much about it. It is experiential and that is why Rolfing cannot be learned from a book. It must be experienced to be transmitted.

In my notes from a class with Tom Wing appear the following words under the heading "key words": Length / extension / lift / space / resilience / freedom / independence / balance / integration.[2] These words touch well on the feeling one is attempting to evoke in the structure and being of the client. This can all be seen in the bodily structure (with much practice) as well as felt in the energy field of the client during and after the process of Rolfing. These words represent the core goals of Rolfing that are implied in the more specific anatomical goals that are addressed in each of the sessions.

I sing of skin, layered fine as baklava, whose colors shame the dawn, at once the scabbard upon which is writ our only signature, and instrument by which we are thrilled. Protected and kept constant in our natural place.

– RICHARD SELZER, MORTAL LESSONS, 105.

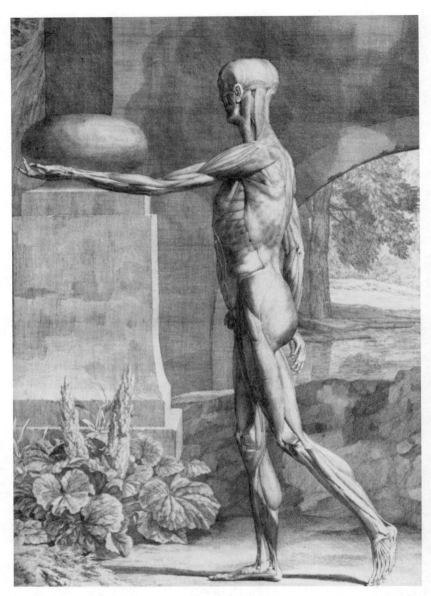

Figure 5.6
"The Outermost Order of Muscles, Side View," from Albinus on Anatomy
by Robert Beverly Hale and Terence Coyle.
Used with permission.

Breathing and the 12ᵗʰ Rib

A key to more open breathing is freeing the tissue around the area of the 12ᵗʰ rib and balancing the quadratus lumborum muscle, which is just posterior to the psoas muscle, which in turn interdigitates with the crurae of the diaphragm. The 12ᵗʰ rib is not attached to costal cartilage and thus has a great deal of possibility for movement. I remember hearing in class that Dr. Rolf was once asked which part of the body she felt was the most important. Her reply was: "If I were to choose a part of the body in which to specialize (heaven forbid!) I would choose the 12ᵗʰ rib. It is involved with respiration, digestion, elimination, and reproduction."[4]

* * *

So far we have brought some length into the torso, worked with the relationship of the torso to the pelvis, and begun to get some differentiation of the thigh from the pelvis. We have kept an eye toward bringing the pelvis toward a more horizontal position over feet that are more grounded and balanced. The superficial fascia of the body has been touched on, and as the outer wrapping of muscles releases, space is created for changes to happen at deeper levels. More open breathing is energizing all the tissues and organs of the body, helping the whole physical system to become more resilient. Length has been created through the muscles of the back and neck, allowing enough space for a more normal C-curve in the spine.

Fascia supports and lifts weight. Weight goes up not down. Bones do not carry weight.

– IDA P. ROLF

The "Core" Hours – Sessions 4-7

The next four sessions, which work deep in the body, are called "core" hours. We begin to work more specifically in the structure with the underlying aberrant patterns in the legs, pelvis, thorax, neck and head. These sessions involve a constant shifting of vision from very specific work to work that integrates and relates the parts – that releases one area in preparation to release the next area, while keeping a feel for the whole system.

As I work, inwardly I am constantly asking questions: "I see the whole pattern. Now how can I take it apart a bit? How can I open some space here, so I can untwist over there, so these pieces can relate to each other in a new way?" All this is considered while keeping track of the client's verbal, energetic, kinesthetic, physical and emotional responses. Sometimes, depending on the client, it's quite a juggling act. This is what makes Rolfing fun and keeps the practitioner awake.

Early in my practice I had a difficult time relating what I saw when clients were standing, to what I saw when they were moving or lying down. If I saw a particular pattern as a whole when they were standing, I had to keep that in mind as I worked specifically and deeply in one area of the pattern. Sometimes a visible change would happen in a specific area when they were lying down, and when they stood and moved I had to reorient my vision to relate how the shifts manifested between those different positions.

After having established some space and length in the outer layers of the body, we begin to look at the inside lines of which Dr. Rolf speaks (*see* sidebar quote). We look specifically now at the adductors and how they are related to the ramus of the ischium. Sometimes the entire inside line from the medial malleolus through the psoas to the back of the diaphragm looks too short – there is an asymmetry of inner to outer lateral line. Two major things to observe: does the pelvic floor look as though it is tilted anterior, or does the pelvic floor look as though it is sucked up toward the abdomen.

In my notes from Tom Wing's class, some of the goals of beginning to establish this inner line are stated in these images:

Meditate on the inside lines of your body. Picture, visualize and do your movements at the intrinsic or bone level.

– IDA P. ROLF

- Establish a line from ramus of the ischium to the ankle.
- Establish span of the adductors.
- Open the inner channel so the psoas can span.
- The leg should let out of the pelvis and lengthen with movement.[5]

The challenge for the Rolfer is to actually manifest such ideas in the flesh and the being of the client, keeping in mind that Dr. Rolf would say: "The ramus of the ischium is the port of entry into the harbor of good tone in the pelvic floor." And, "...the pelvic floor is that area that gathers evolutionary change."[6] As we work, we hold the realization that the inner thigh is often emotionally loaded and can bring up sexual issues. Along with this recognition, the Rolfer will stir in a liberal helping of knowledge of anatomy and top it off with a keen awareness of the client's history and emotional state. Only then is the Rolfer ready to "roll up your sleeves and get to work," as Dr. Rolf would say.

Wow! Sometimes I wonder how we all managed to learn this. But learn it we did – on all channels of awareness combining seeing, touching, being touched, intuition, concrete information, and the magic of the space that was set up by our Rolf teachers within the lineage of Dr. Rolf. Then it was, and is: use your vision and practice, practice, practice.

We would follow this rather enigmatic path that our teachers had laid out for us, and lo and behold, the clients would change, and we would change. The whole process reminded me of my father's egg trick (*see* sidebar), which used to amaze me as a child. I later learned to perform this myself, which was always a hit at any gathering. If you follow the directions exactly, the trick works and in the process you learn to understand the principles behind it.

The same could be said of Rolfing. If you follow the directions of each of the hours in the Ten-Series Recipe you learn to

DAD'S EGG TRICK
Directions
1. *Put a large glass of water at just the right distance from the edge of a counter.*
2. *Place a tin pie plate on top of glass, centering it as much as possible.*
3. *Place up ended small matchbox in center of pie plate lined up with center of glass.*
4. *Place an egg on the matchbox (preferably uncooked – it's more dramatic that way)*
5. *Take a broom and stand on the bent back bristles.*
6. *Bend back the broom handle and aim it toward the glass.*
7. *Let go of the broom handle.*
Result:
Bam! The broom handle hits the counter, the pie plate goes sailing, making a nice crash, and the egg drops neatly into the glass of water (most of the time).

understand the principles. Then, after time and practice, you can work in the territory without the map.

Psoas Muscle (See Figure 5.7)

Only after four hours of previous Rolfing work do we attempt to work directly with the psoas muscle. Balance and relationship between the rectus abdominus and the psoas, and the piriformis and the psoas are keys to relieving low back pain by establishing a horizontal pelvis. (*See* Figure 5.8 on page 84) Without having lengthened the inner line of the thigh from the medial malleolus to the pelvic floor, the attachment of the psoas on the lesser trochanter of the femur would not be free to lengthen. A properly working psoas actually lifts the lumbars posterior and initiates hip flexion. This can be observed in watching someone walk: movement goes through the pelvis instead of around it, and you can see the subtle movement of the lumbars forward and back.

Dr. Rolf considered the psoas to be a muscle that is a key to the evolution of the human from four legged to upright. As stated in her quote above, she felt that no one who hadn't been Rolfed had a psoas that functioned the way she saw and felt it should. To come to a true upright position, you need a properly functioning psoas as well as enough length in the area of the femoral triangle to be able to balance the trunk over the pelvis and have the legs able to freely extend when walking.

Dr. Rolf used to demonstrate the psoas action in her classes, and Peter Melchior described this demonstration:

> She had these little Birkenstocks that fit fairly loosely and she would kick her foot using the quadriceps muscle and nothing would happen. The shoe would still be on her foot. And then she'd start it with the psoas and flip the shoe across the room.[7]

A properly working psoas falls back as you flex the trunk. This is the basic difference between a normal body and a random one. I have never seen a psoas function like this in an unprocessed body.

— IDA P. ROLF

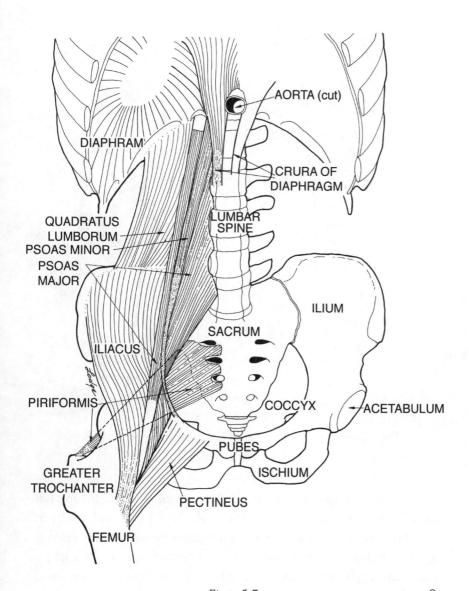

Figure 5.7

The psoas

From Rolfing: The Integration of Human Structures *by Ida P. Rolf.*

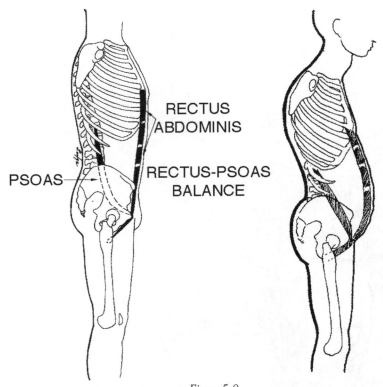

Figure 5.8
The psoas / rectus balance
From Rolfing: The Integration of Human Structures *by Ida P. Rolf.*
Used with permission.

This action of the psoas is also important for establishing balanced secondary curves of the spine. A short psoas and a forward tilted pelvis with an exaggerated lumbar curve will usually encourage a matching exaggerated secondary cervical curve. In a lateral curvature of the spine (or scoliosis) one psoas muscle is shortened, as is shown in Figure 5.9. I remember that once during a class I was having a terrible time seeing. My vision felt blurry and I felt sleepy and foggy as though I couldn't stay awake. My Rolf teacher,

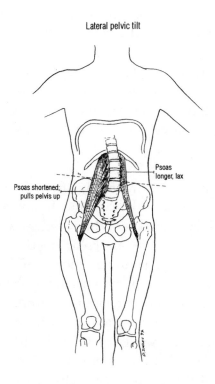

Figure 5.9
Psoas with scoliosis
From The Endless Web *by R. Louis Schultz, Ph.D. and Rosemary Feitis, D.O.*
Used with permission.

Emmett Hutchins, sat me down on a bench and began to work on my psoas as I leaned forward and back from the hip joint. By working with me sitting and moving, he was able to go deep, but still keep integration. Also, since I had had extensive Rolfing, there was enough space to enable him to directly access my psoas. As we began to establish more lift and length in my psoas, a pull that had been happening at my 3rd cervical vertebra began to release. With only five minutes of neck work and an integrating pelvic lift, I felt like someone had turned on the lights and I was awake again.

> If a body is normal, the psoas should elongate during flexion and fall back toward the spine...By virtue of this, the normal psoas forms an important part of a supporting web holding the lumbar vertebrae appropriately spanned.
>
> – Ida P. Rolf[8]

The rectus abdominus muscle is often shortened along its course between the area of the costal arch and pubic symphysis. Overuse and over development of this muscle as a result of certain types of body conditioning lessens psoas function by not allowing it enough space for its full spanning action. This is one of the purposes of working first to loosen patterns in the abdominal obliques and rectus abdominus before attempting to work on the psoas.

Working once with a medical doctor, he was quite shocked when I mentioned that I was going to work with the psoas, as he had an intricate knowledge of anatomy and physiology. *How do you get through all the organs and muscles that are in front of the psoas?* Good question. You work slowly, with great sensitivity, and with proper angle of the fingers. Amazingly, you can feel the psoas pop out under your fingers when your client gently bends his knee and takes his foot a little off the bed. Great sensitivity of touch is required for working appropriately in the abdominal area. It has taken four previous sessions of work to bring the body to a level of resilience and space that allows for working on these deeper structures.

Although I am not specifically trained to feel organs in the body, I have occasionally felt tumors. With one woman I felt a mass almost as big as a grapefruit that later turned out to be a benign uterine tumor. She had no awareness that it was there. The first time I put my hands into the abdominal tissue little red lights went on in my brain as it didn't feel like normal connective tissue. When I called her attention to it, she too was able to feel it. I suggested that she get her doctor to check it, which is how we discovered that it was a uterine tumor, luckily benign.

Rotations of the Femur

At last we get to work with rotations of the femur, which we have been noticing all along. The work to release and align the heels from earlier hours creates the base we need to begin to establish sacral respiration. The work to balance the pelvic floor establishes an entryway to balance the coccyx. The lengthening of the psoas gives space to address the sacrum and its relationship to the ilium and spine.

Rotations of the femur can be addressed by working at the back of the lesser trochanter of the femur where the deep outward rotators attach and then span from there to the sacrum. Each of the previous sessions have set up the possibility for the femur to move freely, independent of the pelvis, and especially for the hamstrings to lengthen when the thigh is brought forward.

The hamstrings must be lengthened around their attachments at the ischial tuberosity before the deep outward rotators of the thigh can be addressed. In Figure 5.10 you will see quite an intricate group of muscles attaching on the greater trochanter of the femur, with hamstrings attaching on the ischial tuberosity and gluteus maximus crossing over the top. One of the key muscles in this group is the piriformis muscle. "This muscle extends from the anterior aspect of the middle of the sacrum to the upper border of the greater trochanter. It emerges from the pelvis through the greater sciatic foramen. Within the pelvis it lies posterior to the sacral plexus."[9] The nerve roots at the 4th and 5th lumbar vertebrae join with the upper three sacral nerves to form the sacral plexus. From most of this plexus the sciatic nerve forms and passes through the greater sciatic foramen to innervate the gluteal region

The body says what words cannot.
– MARTHA GRAHAM

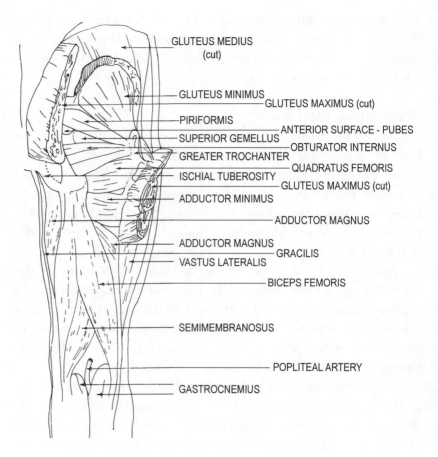

Figure 5.10
Outward rotators
From Rolfing: The Integration of Human Structures *by Ida P. Rolf.*
Used with permission.

and the posterior thigh.[10] Common sciatic pain in the general hip region often has to do with a tight piriformis that is literally con-stricting the sciatic nerve as it passes through the greater sciatic foramen and on down the back of the leg. The piriformis and psoas are two muscles that are often related to back pain and sciatic pain, but they are two of the deepest muscles in the body and much space and length has been created before directly addressing these muscles.

The Coccyx

The coccyx is somewhat like the 11th and 12th ribs in that it has only one point of anchorage. All those falls on the butt can knock the coccyx every which way. I have felt the coccyx in all manner of surprising positions. Just in front of the coccyx is the Ganglion of Impar. As I learned from Emmett Hutchins:

> The "secret doctrine" of yoga deals with the Ganglion of Impar. This ganglion is the lowest in the chain of autonomic plexi, having cells in common with the central nervous system and both halves of the autonomic nervous system. Both sympathetic and motor systems can be balanced and controlled through the Ganglion of Impar. It also has much to do with the regulation of blood pressure throughout the body.[11]

Emmett had more to say about the importance of balancing the coccyx, as I noted from his class: In Hindu medical practice this Ganglion of Impar was considered the seat of the soul. You can regulate the heart from stimulation of the Ganglion of Impar. There is a matching ganglion deep in the tissues of the nose called the Ganglion of Ribes, which also has cells in common with the central and autonomic nervous systems. Both of these ganglia are involved with the esoteric channels of *ida*, *pingala* and *sushumna*, which are affected in the breathing practices of *pranayama*. Perhaps these ganglia can be directly affected by the practice of *pranayama*, and may be how yogis are able to control autonomic functions such as the regulation of the heart.[12]

At this point in my practitioner training I was struggling with my own relationship between the spiritual and the material. I was at the time connected with Swami Amar Jyoti, a Vedantic East Indian spiritual teacher. Before he suggested that I become a Rolfer and I ventured on this path, I was aspiring to leave the world behind. I thought I was on the spiritual path to be free of suffering, to escape the world by entering into nirvana. But guess who suggested I take the path of Rolfing, a path grounded in physical reality? That very same spiritual teacher.

I remember lying face down on the table in the Rolfing room at the old Pearl Street Rolf Institute. My class partner was working around my sacrum and I remember feeling as though I wasn't sure I wanted to change anymore. In a way that I didn't know at the time, my old belief system that you could never realize God here in a human body was being slowly dismantled. Looking back, I see the tremendous wisdom in my spiritual teacher's suggestion, which involved the whole journey of coming into groundedness and relationship with the earth – with where I am and who I am.

You create a different person by re-organizing the head in space.
– IDA P. ROLF

The Head

The head – "mission control" – the upper pole! During my practitioner training, on the day in 1978 when we began to study the head, I remember the group of us camped near the skeleton poking around in the jaw and cranium, looking at the structure of the nose, and flipping through our anatomy books. After doing our best to establish a horizontal pelvis beneath it, my class partner and I were about to get to work to learn about changing structure in the head and neck area.

We began to look at the relationship of the neck to the thorax, the head to the neck, and the balance of the sphenoid bone. As I was going to give my partner the session first, I watched her turn her head right and left, and nod up and down to notice if there was even movement to both sides, and whether the spine

turned without dragging on the clavicle or rest of the shoulder girdle. I began to see the head and spine as one unit separate from the
shoulder girdle, and to look at the eyes and imagine the balance of
the sphenoid bone. For the last six sessions we had been building
the length, space, and base of support to finally be able to address
getting the head to rest horizontally on top of a horizontal pelvis.
We had worked to get the sacrum to relate to the spine over the
more balanced heels we had established in earlier hours. The deep
muscles of the psoas and piriformis were more related, bringing
more right left balance to the pelvis. Now it was time for me to
work on, as Ida would say, "putting the head on."

Before we go "bopping" into the core of someone's head, again
there is much preparation. There are three layers of muscles that
cross the atlanto-occipital joint and attach on the occiput. They
are responsible for varying degrees of extension, rotation, and side
bending of the head on the neck.[13] All the nerves and blood vessels to the brain and head pass through the neck. One look at dia-
grams of the deep layers of the neck in an anatomy text is enough
to bring one to sobriety regarding the care and sensitivity of touch
that is required. One must swim through the tissues with fingers
alive to every response and feeling of what is under them. We can
reach the surface layers of trapezius, sternocleidomastoid, platys-
ma, and nuchal ligament directly. More experienced Rolfers can
work with splenius capitus, scalenes, and levator scapulae if we
stay awake to our client's responses. The deepest muscles of the
neck such as the prevertebral muscles are reached by intention.

Work on the anterior neck, other then the superficial muscles,
is generally not taught in basic Rolf classes. It was only after many
hours of four-handed work with Emmett Hutchins – working in
the area of sternocleidomastoid, scalenes, and levator scapulae,
while I held the back of the client's head and felt the shifts
between our four hands – that I had a sense of what could be done
with the proper knowledge. Later, when Stacey Mills (a senior

*The brain is the largest
nerve center in the body
and putting the head on
will change your entire
gait.*

– IDA P. ROLF

Rolf teacher) was staying with me in Boulder while she taught a class, I received quite a bit of neck and head work from her. From my own awareness of receiving and watching those sessions I began to learn how to work on specific muscles of the anterior neck. This adds a new dimension to working with the cervical curve (or lack of it). The cervical curve and the lumbar curve are related, and just as length in the psoas allows the lumbars to lift posterior, lengthening the muscles in the front of the neck will help to balance the cervical curve.

After having brought some length and resilience to the areas of upper ribs and neck we can move on to addressing the head directly. If we plan to work in the jaw, palate, and nose, we first loosen the fascial "bathing cap" of the cranium where the neck and facial muscles attach. The work inside the mouth is powerful and can elicit profound changes in the craniosacral rhythm, as well as shift curvatures in the spine. The sphenoid bone is the deepest and most central part of the cranium, and we can actually affect its balance through the work on the medial and lateral pterygoids as well as directly on the hard palate, which is the base of the sphenoid. The sphenoid bone is the key to balancing the head.

Any imbalance in the pelvis and/or spine will end up reflecting in the hard palate. As Jan Sultan mentioned, and I recorded in my class notes, sometimes chronic asthma or bronchitis will alter the shape of the palate. The shape of the palate affects the bony relationships of the cranium.[14] Again, it is possible to actually change the shape of the palate, thus it is important to ask the client if he or she is wearing dentures, braces, or is in the process of other dental repair work. By changing the palate, the fit of the dentures may also change. This could be positive or negative for the client.

We finally approach the hidden treasure deep in the cave of the cranium – the sphenoid bone itself, reached by way of the medial pterygoid. When contacting the medial pterygoid muscles I have often felt a gentle watery wave of release coursing from the center of the head down to the pelvis. If there is an imbalance in the pelvis, I will often find one medial pterygoid shorter or in a different position than the other, much like you would find in the psoas. Not enough can be said on the care one must take with the client through this process. Often, past trauma will come up in this session. Watching closely for autonomic responses and stopping to give space for these responses to cycle through, will often save a big emotional reaction from happening (though not always). More on this is covered in Chapter 11, *Trauma*.

After this attention to the sphenoid it is the time to consider the nose work, if the client needs it and wants "The Full Monty." People who are habitual mouth breathers, have a deviated septum, have allergies, or have trouble breathing through the nose can often receive considerable relief from work inside the nose.

The other nerve ganglion that matches the Ganglion of Impar is the Ganglion of Ribes which can be affected by work in the nose. This ganglion is not mentioned in Western anatomy texts. In my interview with Jeff Linn, the archivist of Dr. Rolf's tapes, he described his knowledge of the Ganglion of Ribes as follows:

> What I know about Ribes is Ribes is a near mystical ganglion. If you find an anatomy book that talks about it, they basically talk about the terminus of autonomic fibers snaking their way up along the carotid arteries and then ultimately terminating at the anterior communicating artery which joins the two sides of the arterial cerebral flow at the circle of Willis...so it comes up and follows this up on the circle of Willis and then lands on the anterior communicating artery which is real close to the sella turcica on the sphenoid.[15]

Ida and Pingala nerve centers inside the nose are extremely important to mental and physical health. Both halves of the nose must balance.
— IDA P. ROLF

I don't suppose many of us think about tension in our nose. But we can and do tense our noses, as strange as that might seem, and this does have an effect on the way we breathe. The little rounded bumps on the sides of your nose are called wings (alae, singular ala). These wings should be soft and passive during both quiet breathing and pranayama.

— RICHARD ROSEN, THE YOGA OF BREATH, 116.

Linn thinks Dr. Rolf may have learned about this from a particular chiropractor. She may also have learned it from her study of yoga.

I once found an old yoga book by an East Indian author when I was poking around in an ashram library looking for books on *pranayama*, the science of breath. I remember being quite surprised to read about all the negative points of habitual breathing through the mouth. Breathing through the nose activates the subtle movement of the cranial bones, filters dust and airborne particles, as well as warms cold air coming into the lungs. I also remember reading that a good Ayurvedic doctor could diagnose certain pathologies by noticing which nostril was most open at what time of day.

I do not always do the nose work in the basic Ten Series except when the client indicates a particular need for it or interest in having more open breathing through the nose. I always explain what I am going to do and why, and give the client the option to go forward with it or not. By this time we've been working with each other for six previous hours and have a certain trust and rapport with each other. Many clients report that the nose work helped them enough so that they ask me to work in their nose again in later hours.

As I approached my practitioner training, I realized that I had never had the nose work done, as my Rolfer's hands were too big. Since I was going to be required to give and receive this work in class I signed up for an hour of Rolfing with Tom Wing, a Rolf Instructor, senior Rolfer, and assistant at that time in my class. Tom is so kind, so supportive, so *with* you, that I often feel that in getting Rolfed by him I change because he sees and relates to who I *could* be – my highest self. That was one wild hour! I had so much old trauma stored in my head, jaw and nose that I cried buckets, my nose bled all over Tom's Rolfing bed, and I probably got snot everywhere. Thankfully, Tom was right there with me through it all. Afterward, I felt totally altered. The openness of breath through my nose and the new balance in my head gave me a different perception of the world. I remember walking on the Boulder Mall and thinking that everything I saw was part of a movie set. Things seemed to have less substance and density as though I was seeing reality in a deeper way. The combination of being grounded in physical reality while walking through a level of illusion was something I had never experienced before. Needless to say, after having experienced the power of that session on my head, I was wide awake to being sensitive to my class partner in our exchange of sessions.

* * *

At this point in the Rolfing sessions we have climbed the mountain from the feet to the head and reached some of the deepest structures in the body. Now, the experiences of the mountaintop must be integrated into three-dimensional reality. After enlightenment we still chop wood and carry water, as the old Zen saying goes.

The last fifteen minutes or so of any "head hour" is to integrate the changes in the head and neck all the way down through the body and into the feet. As the client first sits and then stands, I make sure she has her eyes open and clear and has her feet well grounded on the floor. I might use some of the eye-integrating exercises mentioned next. I often tell the client to walk outside a bit before getting in the car to drive home. There is a new reality to integrate – a lift through the top of the head while being grounded through the feet.

The Eyes and Alignment

The eyes are important in establishing kinesthetic center around the spine. As a standard anatomy text states: "There are a large number of small muscles between the atlas, axis and occipital bone. This is associated with the small adjustments of the position of the head connected with the movements of the eyes."[16]

With the client sitting, and finding the top of his head in his inner awareness, I rest my fingers lightly on top of the client's head and feel, with my awareness, down the two sides of the body on the inside to the sit bones. I then ask the client if he feels that each eye is lined up over each sit bone. I can feel him make little adjustments through the body. Then I ask the client to feel the palate and find the way out of the top of his head from there. Then he can ground his feet, finding awareness in his body from feet to sit bones to palate to top of the head. Having him keep his eyes open while doing this keeps him present in this here and now. Sometimes I have had clients feel not quite present at the end of the session, especially where there have been shifts in the spine. Working gently with the eyes and their relationship around the spine usually clears this up quickly.

The more head that exists in back of the ears, the less ego involved. – Emmett Hutchins[17]

I threw in this above quote just to get your attention!

Looking at a skeleton from the side, you see that there is about as much mass behind the region of the ear as in front. Yet often, you see heads carried forward, with the neck muscles pulled forward, and more energy and awareness in the front of the head than in the back. Close use of the eyes – such as happens if the client does a lot of reading or computer work – pulls the energy forward into the face. The eyes then "reach out" to see, as opposed to allowing information to be received. I think one of the best balanced head and neck structures I've ever seen in an un-Rolfed person is the little Bushman who stars in the film "The Gods Must Be Crazy." A lifetime of the kind of distance gazing done by indigenous people

I suspect that this universal life force may well be another name for God, or the universal creator. And I believe that God, therefore, exists within all of us, embodied in this energy. Most people today have been schooled to believe that God exists without, rather than within themselves. I think this is a mistake. Certainly, if you believe that God is within, you will start to take much better care of your body, for your body truly is your temple.

– ROBERT FULFORD, D.O.

who are hunters and trackers uses more of the intuitive centers in the back of the head. When the head is horizontal and directly over the pelvis, the eyes have the opportunity to relax and gaze straight forward, as if they originated in the back of the head. (*See* Figure 5.11)

I once took a class from Rosemary Feitis who had studied with Dr. Amos Gunsberg, a performance coach who had an innate ability to see into the brain. She was studying a particular way to access deep awareness through coaching a partner to drop deeper into the brain by using his or her eyes as indicators. Rosemary in

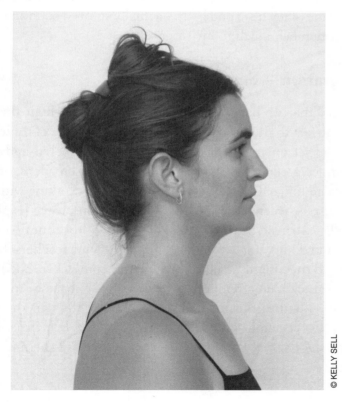

© KELLY SELL

Figure 5.11
Side view of head

turn was teaching this to our group of Rolfers. We were learning to allow our awareness to drop back into the center of the brain so that information would come in without always being filtered through the previous information, like a film being wound back after each picture. At the time, we were in the dome room at the Rolf Institute on Pearl Street in Boulder. A small fenced courtyard could be seen through the room's sliding glass doors. In one exercise, we were to stand with our backs to the courtyard and count off the number of posts on the fence by intending to see out of the back of our heads. I remember standing there counting the posts and feeling like I just knew where they were by focusing on the back plane of my head and body. I actually stopped counting at the correct number, much to my surprise.

Integration – Sessions 8-10

Now that we have made some changes throughout the body from the feet to the head, we can go back over some of those same areas and get a higher level of organization of the pelvic and shoulder girdles around the spine. Here our vision broadens, and we look more for goals in movement. We are now working with relationships: between structure and function, core/sleeve [explained below], extrinsic/intrinsic, inside/outside, horizontal/vertical, being and doing. It is my understanding from my teachers that Dr. Rolf used these terms, especially the terms core/sleeve, and intrinsic/extrinsic, in an attempt to explain a level of balance involving specific polarities that related to each other through the single organizing principle of the Rolf Line. In *Ida Rolf Talks About Rolfing and Physical Reality* she uses an example of the muscles of the neck.

The outer muscles of the neck function as a bandage. They bind the head to the trunk. In my own opinion, and this is

Work *is the job of the sleeve*, being *is the job of the core. When these are not kept separate, trouble and fatigue ensue.*

– IDA P. ROLF

pure and unadulterated opinion, those outer muscles that go from head to shoulder are not intended for rotation. They adjust to rotation, but I think the neck is designed so that the function of rotation is taken on by the intrinsics (the deep short muscles) of the neck. If the head is too far forward, rotation is done by the extrinsics because the intrinsics then lack span and can't function, but to the extent that this happens, the normal patterning of the body is destroyed. The balanced core and sleeve pattern of the body gets lost.[18]

Rosemary Feitis, the editor of *Ida Rolf Talks*, describes Dr. Rolf's use of the terms intrinsic/extrinsic as follows:

As used by Dr. Rolf, "intrinsic" and "extrinsic" are functional categories. The rule of thumb is that tissue nearer the bone is intrinsic, tissue closer to the surface is extrinsic. In terms of movement, intrinsics will initiate a movement, extrinsics will take it further…Intrinsic movement as a whole is initiated from the core of the body, most probably by the older vegetative autonomic nervous system.[19]

In my class notes I find that all four of my teachers mentioned that Dr. Rolf used the terms "core/sleeve" as a metaphor to define inside/outside symmetry and relationship. The trunk of the body was referred to as the "core," and the pelvic and shoulder girdles were referred to as the "sleeve." The idea was to see movement that began in the core of the body with the feeling that the shoulder and pelvic girdles were not impinging on the core. Feitis put it well when she said: "The girdles (shoulder and pelvic) express the will of the being – they *do*, but in doing they should be sufficiently free so that their actions do not distort the serenity of the core."[20] Whenever I see movement that demonstrates this (which is rarely), it catches my attention with the feeling of effortless grace and flow.

Being and *doing*...how do we manage that? Perhaps only in considering the concept and holding it as a question while we work. This relationship between being and doing is no small thing. For me it is a lifetime exploration. I feel the principle of this metaphor most when I am physically relaxed but not collapsed. When I am doing a job such as covering a bank of dirt with carefully placed river stones, I can slow down and watch my movements and thoughts. Such a job has a clearly progress-oriented goal, yet it can also be meditative. It is tempting to think that being can only be felt in stillness and doing only in action. I have surely felt action when sitting in meditation and relaxation of mind when doing a physical job.

A Rolfer must first learn to separate an intrinsic movement from an extrinsic one in order to begin to unscramble stuck patterns and experience what an intrinsic movement feels like before she can evoke this in her client. "Deep," "slow," "small," and "wavelike" are descriptions of intrinsic movement. "Surface," "fast," "large," and "sharp" are more extrinsic. Many people are moving so fast and with so much tension in their lives that they have rarely if ever experienced that deep, slow, wavelike kind of movement. We have to teach them, and there are many opportunities to do this as we process through the Rolfing.

I might ask a client to do a gentle movement, a small flexion of the knee for example. She will often do a large movement involving many more muscles than are needed. Yet, if I suggest that she just imagine moving her knee, she will make a much more subtle movement, and this can begin to give her the feeling that she doesn't need to work as hard. It can also be frustrating to someone who is used to moving quickly and superficially, so time and patience are needed.

You cannot experience true joint movement until it is initiated from the inside with intrinsic muscles. Any movement which is primarily extrinsic is only an approximation of true movement.

— IDA P. ROLF

When working with the pelvic girdle we will look at the inner and outer suspension lines of the pelvis and legs. The inner suspension of psoas, iliacus, and adductors down to the medial arch of the foot is where movement should originate. (*See* Figure 5.12) For stability we look at the outer suspension of the lumbar fascia, the outward rotators of the thigh, the iliotibial tract down to the outer arch of the foot. When these two lines of suspension are working well there is a flow of movement that involves the psoas muscle when the person is walking. Even though we are again considering the psoas, we are looking with broader vision and less specificity than the first time we touched on the psoas.

Emmett Hutchins often suggested that we find a safe space and walk backwards, which was a way to connect with not only the psoas, but also the backside of the body and the heel. We used to try this on the beach in Kauai when I was there assisting Emmett with an advanced Rolfing class. We must have looked rather unusual; the whole group of us walking backwards down the beach. When there is plenty of space and you feel that you don't have to keep looking over your shoulder, there is a wonderful connection to the heel as it reaches back with the backward stride. It was fun feeling the backside of the body for a change too. If you can separate the front from the back, then you can find the middle where you really live. I once suggested this backward walking to an enthusiastic and dedicated client. She came back the next week and told me that she had been walking backward along the main street in the little town where she lived and had been stopped by a policeman and told to cease and desist as it was too dangerous. I guess it wasn't a very high crime town!

When working with the shoulder girdle we look also for a balance between inner and outer suspension. The inner line goes from the palms of the hands up the insides of the arms through the armpit, into the throat and front of the neck and jaw. The outer line consists of the lateral arch of the hand to the outside of the

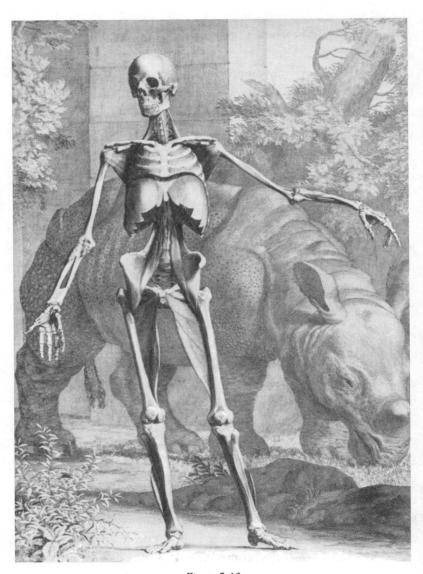

Figure 5.12
"The Fourth Order of Muscles, Front View"
From Albinus on Anatomy *by Robert Beverly Hale and Terence Coyle.*
Used with permission.

arms, to the rhomboids, teres muscles, to the back of the neck and head. The arms are especially expressive, and the support of an aligned and dynamic pelvic girdle allows for the client's exploration and development of her expansion and creativity.

Ron McComb, a long-time Rolfer and student of Dr. Rolf's, suggests a deep connection between the emotions and the arms:

> Today I am able to put into words a discovery arising out of a long held suspicion that there is a strong connection between the hands and the core through the emotions. That is, that the hands are an extension of the ego. The hands protect the core and give it nourishment. Tight forearms defend the heart continuously, whereas open forearms and hands are disconnected from the ego and are connected, or are an extension of the heart, such as in the repose of the hands of the Buddha. Instead of moving compulsively from the ego, the hands wait to be moved by the heart.

Dr. Rolf had a specific way that she felt the arms should hang if the shoulder girdle was properly balanced; that is, with the elbow facing outward from the side of the body. The shoulder should release and the arm lengthen with an intrinsic movement of the elbows out. For most people this is a foreign movement, and you can watch the client use a lot of extrinsic movement in the shoulder girdle to try to accomplish this. If the shoulder girdle is rolled even slightly forward, the rhomboids disengage and the front of the shoulder does more of the work. I've only seen one person who had that natural movement without having been Rolfed and that was Swamiji, my first spiritual teacher. He was East Indian and a lifelong yoga practitioner. He had one of the most beautifully balanced shoulder girdle, neck, and head structures I've ever seen. When he walked, his arms didn't swing much from side to side, but bobbed gently up and down at the elbow

Cautiousness is measured by the 4th finger. A bold person will have the 4th finger longer than the index finger.

         – IDA P. ROLF

When hands are stiff it means bad arteries and the consumption of too much cholesterol.

         – IDA P. ROLF

If the side of the thumb is blue, there is trouble with digestion.

         – IDA P. ROLF

joint. There was an easy lift through the top of his head. I always had the feeling that his walk was neither too fast nor too slow; the rhythm of it was remarkable to me and when I would hear him walking outside on the gravel driveway, there was no mistaking who it was.

> The condition of the shoulder girdle always reflects the condition of the arms. As you let out tension in the forearms, the shoulders begin to change and then the thorax changes via the pectoral attachments. – Ida P. Rolf[21]

Freeing the knots in the forearms and opening the inner and outer arches of the hands can do wonders at releasing the shoulder girdle and neck, as Dr. Rolf has stated above. I learned much about the power of working on the hands and arms from working four-handed with Emmett Hutchins during the time I lived in Boulder. I could feel all kinds of "pool shots" of movement and change projecting from his hands, through the client's body, to mine. I learned that there is always another end to the problem on which you are working. Some of these connections might be hard to find in an anatomy book, or with linear, cause-and-effect thinking, but I certainly could *feel* things shifting when the three of us were hooked in together. These relationships are what we are beginning to establish in these later sessions.

The functional/experiential core is the psoas/rhomboid balance. The physiological core is the psoas/diaphragm relationship.
— IDA P. ROLF

The Last Hour

> Perfection is the remedy for linear problems and life is circular. – Ida P. Rolf

> We are evolving creatures. We are not trying to go back to some perfect state. – Ida P. Rolf

The ideas expressed in these words of Ida Rolf must be kept in mind as we do the last hour in the Ten-Session Series. This hour is about closure to the journey we have taken with our client. The client knows from the beginning that we will work together for ten hours and then they will be on their own for awhile to integrate and enjoy all that has happened.

In some ways the tenth hour is more mysterious than any of the others. The key is to work with large fascial planes in order to bring horizontals into the flesh. This does not happen without the previous nine hours. It is extremely tempting to spend the hour trying to "fix" something that isn't quite how you'd like to see it. Maybe the pelvis isn't totally horizontal, or the spinal twist you've been working with is still there to some degree. You have to let go and realize that this is as far as you have gotten. Not only is your client making closure with you, but you are also making closure with the client. It's a good place to practice karma yoga – do your best and release the results. Still, a lot can happen in the tenth hour if you know what things to leave undone, and what things to do.

The whole body should be one complete interrelated whole. Usually, just one or two moves in an area is enough to make it change easily. Anything that does not change easily is not ready to change. The tissue should feel silky and soft. This is not the time for deep work to try to open up something new, but a time to balance all the changes we've gotten so far.

I usually find the tenth session to be easy and enjoyable, both for the client and myself and he or she usually feels grounded, yet light, with a feeling of integration and an ease of movement. I don't think I can ever remember a client having problems, or an emotional outburst or trauma arising in a tenth session. Such things have come up in some client on every other session but the tenth. The tenth hour embodies our idea about a line of verticality with

Rolfing opens you up to the potentials, and then you have to invest in [this potential] and imbue in it your humanity, your expressiveness. What I have seen with some people who get Rolfed is that they are opened by the Rolfing physically and then because they don't do certain kinds of work that is expressive, gradually it winds back into the old pattern and the flesh re-establishes the blockages that were…broken up by the Rolfer.

— PAUL OERTEL,
DANCER

joints functioning horizontally. It's everything we've been leading up to.

There's a "four-square" look, and the muscles move freely in their fascial envelopes. Everything in the body is up to present time; there is no one area lagging behind. There are no fireworks, either physical or emotional. It's a relatively quiet and uplifting hour. The client should leave feeling high. We are both wrapping things up, working on a proper ending, much like the closing sentence in the paragraph that the chapter about the first Ten Sessions in "the book" of one's experiences in Rolfing.

What Happens Next?

Many of my clients want to know what happens after they have completed the basic Ten-Session Series. I explain that there is a period of integration wherein the changes will continue happening in the body, and that we want to let those shifts play out fully, without immediately interrupting the process with more Rolfing work. I tell the client that he or she will know when it is time for more work: perhaps she will find herself slipping back into old habits; or she wants to work on a chronic situation, or to evolve further into a higher level of organization, or (God forbid) she has had an accident or fall that has thrown her out of alignment. Part of the client's new job of awareness is to know intuitively when she or he is ready for more Rolfing.

A break in any series of Rolfings is also important while the client heightens her ability to notice how she feels, what her daily habit patterns are, and how she is moving through life. We have been working together to help her establish new awareness and new patterns of movement and to be able to recognize and bring to consciousness old stuck patterns that have been harmful. She is thus empowered to take responsibility for growing into the changes she has experienced.

While some people are content with one "chapter" of Rolfing, endless explorations are there for the taking after the basic Ten Sessions. Most will continue to receive Rolfing now and then throughout their lives in the form of a "Three Series" once or twice a year, or a "tune up" session when needed. Clients with a chronic situation often receive many more sessions, as we continue to unravel patterns that may have been lodged in their bodies for ten or twenty years. Rolfing is a process that can continue on in any way that serves the client. With further work the client and I can invent ways for more and deeper change. For some, the more dramatic and noticeable changes happen in advanced work.

Responsibility for continuing along the path toward higher order, or at least for maintaining the changes received, rests with the client. Maintaining the results of Rolfing takes focus and the willingness to change. Luckily, Rolfing affords an increase in awareness. Old habit patterns – such as slouching, always turning in the same direction, sitting with the same leg crossed over the other, favoring an ankle that was once injured, not exercising, eating poorly – can be changed once one is aware of them. Now the client must go out on her own and work with what she has learned and received.

The Teachers Speak about the Ten-Session Series

To add even more mystery to Dr. Rolf's Ten-Session Series Recipe, I asked my teachers about whether they were still using this basic Recipe with people who are new to Rolfing. The answers that follow here are brief – I am sure that each of them could write a book on their feelings, ideas, and experiences regarding this core piece with which Dr. Rolf has challenged us all.

I asked them: How does one use a recipe to learn about the principles hidden within it? What exactly is this so-called Ten-Session Series? Their answers show clearly the divergent paths

Advanced Rolfing at its best and deepest involves real teamwork between the Rolfer and Rolfee. The Rolfer must be able to feel the layering in the body, see and feel upon which layer to work, and engage the Rolfee in new and different ways to find her Line and connect through the area being worked on. The Rolfee must be familiar with and unafraid of intense sensation. She must trust the Rolfer and keep constant focus in her body.

– BETSY SISE

that have been taken. Although all four mention that at some level the principles contained in the Recipe are the core of Rolfing, they each have a different take on how to work to attain such goals in the structure of the body. Ida Rolf, I believe, was a true teacher, and as such she interacted with her students in various and personal ways depending on what each needed. Such teachers will often give students different assignments, and will be paradoxical and often hard to pin down.

These four teachers came from different backgrounds, had different interests, and each had unique experiences of Dr. Rolf. No matter what each of them felt about the Ten Sessions, each developed his own advanced work around his own particular interests and talents.

It is not within the scope of this book to delve into the intricacies of the advanced work, so the following responses of the teachers are focused on the basic Ten Series.

* * *

Emmett Hutchins

"Just before she [Dr. Rolf] died she told me that one of my jobs was to put meaning to the Recipe…she implied that it was a metaphysical kind of thing. She said I should look in Western metaphysics to find my answers…She said several things about the Recipe that were intriguing. One of the many things that I was supposed to figure out was…that the Recipe was a cosmic or eternal kind of sequence, a creation sequence of some kind. She didn't understand it, but she thought it was. If so, then the first three steps held the key to the entire process, not only [to the] ten hours. But you [needed to do] it for a lifetime.

"She said that if I could find the key to the first hour that I would have the key to all the others…I looked for that over and over and over, in every corner…I studied everything that I could.

I couldn't get too far in Kabala because I didn't want to learn Hebrew, but other than that I spent years studying all kinds of things. I found answers in the Yellow Emperor's classic – I didn't just stay with Western metaphysics. But anyway, when I was down in Brazil, in Sao Paulo, about eight years ago, I remember waking up in the morning and sort of meditating for inspiration for the day, and all of a sudden I got this; I knew immediately that the key for the first three hours had just happened. It was almost like I dreamed it in the night and when I woke up I knew!

"I don't claim to feel that this is the complete answer, because I think that the nature of the Recipe is such that it can continue to evolve information forever. But, it was very clear to me that the principle of the first hour, which is the key to everything you do from then on, was the idea of layering. If you are going to start order in the body you start by creating layers; and so the whole idea of the first hour is to create the outside layer. You have to start in the beginning.

"It's taken me my whole career, over thirty-five years, to realize that no matter what I'm doing on what kind of a body, no matter how sophisticated or how new, I'm always working with layers, with the same layer in the knee as I'm working with in the elbow. If I don't work on the same layer in the body then I don't get integration. And that's taken me many many many years to learn.

"So, even though it's a principle of the first session of the basic Ten Series, I think it's one of those things that it takes many years to really master. Ida implied that it was true. If you asked Ida how well a person could do in their first hour she would always say, "Well it depends on how many 10th hours that he does." In other words, you really have to understand the entire process and have it in your being before this idea of layering becomes real.

"Yes, she did mention that she thought that the Recipe and doing this work was an evolutionary path…and that the ritual of that path was the doing of the Ten-Hour Recipe. I have told my classes for years that I think the Recipe is more powerful now than it was back then, because if it is a ritual, and I think it is in some sense, our rituals get more powerful with the repeating. Over the years the more people repeat them, the more power the ritual gets. I've always felt that the Recipe works better, certainly it does for me, now than it did back then, and it works better in general even for beginners. Part of it is this ritual aspect of it. I also believe that it is a growth path, a spiritual growth path, and that it is so even if you don't think it's so. Even if you are into it just for money and business, eventually you are either going to get out of it or it's going to change you. So, I think that it doesn't make any difference whether you believe that or not, it still serves that purpose. It's not necessary to mention [this to students or clients] and I don't think that it's important. I don't require that students have that idea about it because if it truly is the way it is, it doesn't need me to say it to make it that way."

Interviewer: So, as an advanced Rolfer, if you were still working with the general folks you would still use this Ten-Session Series on a person who had never had Rolfing?

Emmett: "Oh of course! I think there is no more efficient way to establish order. It's very clear. If you do a first hour and you can see structure, you see that you must do the second hour, and you see that the second hour must involve the feet, and it must involve some kind of extension.

"The Recipe, as Ida always maintained, writes itself. It isn't something that she invented, it's something she discovered. She hoped that the Recipe would last forever, and she also was definite that it was not to be changed, only to be understood, only to be performed better, to be comprehended better, not to be modified or changed. In my whole lifetime I've not modified it in any way that I know of. I keep my original notes. Every time I teach I go back and look at my original notes to make sure that I haven't gotten too far away or added too much stuff that is my own. I want to keep as much of the original impact of the message as possible.

"She, by the way, did not want any of us to write down the Recipe or to write down lessons to teach the Recipe because she wanted her whole system to be a folk art. She did not want it written down and codified by anybody with authority, so none of her teachers have ever written down the Recipe. She wanted the Recipe to be retold in the idiom of the decade in which it was learned, and she wanted it to grow with the culture, grow with the times, grow with the thinking of the people. [She held] that the Recipe was so basic that it would adapt to any kind of thinking or culture as it went along if you didn't write it down and make it less flexible. So I learned a very flexible but rigid Recipe, and I never deflected from it. But to me it is certainly not confining. It is not a form that prohibits me from doing anything. It only facilitates."

Interviewer: You find that it can be adapted equally to any type of structure?

Emmett: "I think so…I think it never loses its power. Ida implied that the Ten Series should not be repeated more than four or five times on the same individual. If you do it more than that, depending on the structure, you tend to have to create some disorder to get more order. She felt [that with] sophisticated bodies that had gone through that process several times, you ought to be able to work on them without regressing at all. The Recipe sort of does that, if you do the whole ten. She did teach advanced training and advanced work, but the ten never loses its power. For instance, I've worked on people, off and on, not continuously, a little series each year, once or twice for as many as twenty-five or thirty years on the same individual. I can think of two people last year [to whom] I said, "Well, let's try the Ten Series." So, after twenty-five

I've always felt that the kingdom of heaven was within, just as the "Good Book" says. We are so blessed by the fact that there are so many doors to that mansion. I have never felt that Structural Integration was the only door, but it certainly is a grand one and it certainly is one that works, and it's one of the real, true, wonderful connections to spirit and to the world and to enjoyment. It is one of the best processes for integrating the material and the spiritual that I know of.
– EMMETT HUTCHINS

years, [and then] doing the Ten Series [again], they were totally blown away – it was the most wonderful experience of their lives. And these are people who had gotten work from me, and I consider myself fairly good. [They had gotten] a little series and they always have loved the work, but when they got the Ten [again] it was a completely new revelation. So you'll never see me be anything but in awe over the Recipe." – *Interview in Kauai, Hawaii, June 9, 2004.*

Peter Melchior

"For me, the Ten-Session Series is the base on which you build all the later work, whatever you are going to do. Whatever that person's going to do in terms of structural integration either has that base or it does not. When we look at somebody and say, "God, I can't believe that person's actually had the kind of work they say they've had," it's because it's a failure in the Ten-Session Series, almost always. That's my feeling about it.

"It's a glorious kind of a formula. You know, in one sense it's unerring and unvariable, and in another sense it's so broad that you can use it on all kinds of different people in many different ways. You would probably not recognize two adjacent 4th sessions that I was doing. You might not know that they were both the same session because they are dictated by what that person's structure is telling me, but the pattern is there nonetheless."

Interviewer: Are you saying that the general goals that Dr. Rolf set up for the sessions is what you are after, and that how you would go about doing it would be different for each person?

Peter: "Yup. And I think in that exact order. I witnessed that once. I was teaching at Stanford and a group of about half a dozen people came up to me and said, 'We're part of this experimental group and could you work on our bodies – give us an assessment?'

Well, this guy had taken them on and decided to see if the Recipe had to be done in the order that she [Dr. Rolf] had presented it. So he gave them 7th sessions and then he gave them 3rd sessions and then he gave [them 2nd sessions], and that's exactly how they looked – scrambled. There was no order there; the thing we look for and get used to seeing was not there."

Interviewer: After all these years, after thirty-five years of Rolfing, do you still feel that the magic of that basic Recipe is something with which you always begin?

Peter: "Absolutely. As a way to start there isn't any better way; I have not found any better way to start. The minute I do, I'll be doing that. It's a work of genius." – *Interview in Lyons, Colorado, March 4, 2004.*

Jan Sultan

"What happened over time was that I broadened my technique. I still know how to do what I call fascial differentiation – and do, when I see the need for a plane to open or for a set of relationships to really change – but you would say I installed a rheostat in my technique. Of course, as soon as we studied with Upledger [craniosacral therapy], it opened up the other end of the technique spectrum to the very subtle, and established sort of a pole to counterpoint Rolf's basic fascial differentiation technique. So I began to spread my work across that spectrum depending on how I perceived the need of the client. It was a huge shift because Rolf's Recipe…did not acknowledge the state of the client. You did the same thing whether they were big, small, young, old thin, fat – and as soon as I (I say I, because this is about me), but I think we or some of us began to broaden our technique it also meant that we were changing Rolf's basic paradigm, which was that it

Seeing a thing once is better than hearing about it 100 times.
– CHINESE PROVERB

became client centered instead of technique centered. [This was a] huge cultural change from Rolf's basic approach.

"Rolfing [is] being expressed now through so many creative individuals and many of them have their own slant on the work. In terms of what's being taught, I think we still teach the basic systematic differentiation along the lines of the Recipe – that that's the core of Rolfing. And if you don't know how to do that, then either your fix-it work or your psychology stuff is not complete, because you don't create the potential for new patterning."

Interviewer: You still teach that basic Ten-Session Series in your classes?

Jan: "Absolutely! It is a great teaching tool."

Interviewer: How about in your Rolfing private practice? Do you still do the Ten-Session Series for people who are new to Rolfing?

Jan: "Rarely. I usually refer the basic work to other Rolfers."

Interviewer: And what made you shift on that one?

Jan: "Really market demand. Over the years a lot of people came to Rolfing for repair work. I think that there was a huge cultural change, which was partly that in the middle of the human potential movement most of the people who were seeking Rolfing were using it as a tool to develop spiritually and psychologically, to get freed from fixations that may have been bound in the body; so it was an adjunct to psychological work. Lots of people came who were doing meditation and inner journey work, and so they were using Rolfing to get more energy online.

"Then, as the human potential movement got absorbed into the mainstream, Rolfing was sought out by people who were looking

Fundamentally, Rolf said [that] Rolfing is not a job it's a way of life...I think that Rolfing is who I am in that way. It really did change my worldview, fundamentally, both to learn about Rolfing and what it meant to me personally, and also to work with individuals professionally. This has given me a huge education about human nature, which has shaped my view of people [at a deep level.]

– JAN SULTAN

for physical rehabilitation from injuries. And at some point those two things are absolutely overlapped. If you've been wounded and adapted, and then you want to 'grow,' you may have to backtrack and repair what isn't functional, what's not moving right, as a foundation for higher order."

Interviewer: You found a different and better way to do that than the basic Ten-Session Series?

Jan: "Well, having said that – I have. This was actually the first place where I got up against Ida's formulas. I started looking at O legs and X legs – varus and valgus legs (see descriptions and illustrations of these leg patterns in Chapter 9), and wondering why we did the same thing no matter what the pattern was. I began to wonder if you treated an X leg different than an O leg if you would accelerate the potential changes. What I discovered was (when I made my first hypothesis) that the lines of transmission of work force were very different in the two types. I started looking for where the tissue was denser in each type and came up with what I call lines of transmission. What happened was [that] it put new demands on the spine. At that point I realized that if I didn't get a whole lot better at understanding the spine, I had better not be doing the lines of transmission in the legs, because it was putting a demand on the spine to re-compensate. That forced my inquiry into the spinal mechanics. So that X and O [issue] really made me see that there were at least two parallel recipes.

"At some point I realized that X legs went with a whole typology, and O legs went with a polar typology, and I suspect that those were genetically derived. Then, of course, you have mixed types: [for example] internal thorax [and] external legs, and so I had [to] run two parallel recipes. You would use one for external segments and one for internal segments. So at that point the Recipe

Ida Rolf was an absolute pioneer in manual therapy. I think partly because of the breakdown in our own unity, Dr. Rolf's work has been absorbed into the culture as technique...But a lot of people who are practicing deep tissue work or [other] forms of manipulation do not have a clue that Ida Rolf was the person who brought it into being.

— JAN SULTAN

changed a lot for me, and I do teach those changes. The Recipe became more client centered.

"I'm not Rolfing if I don't have gravity in there. But how I do the process in my practice is that I will often look at somebody and think, "Oh this person needs a 4th hour." [They might have] what I would call a '4th hour body' in the sense that the internal [line] from the inside of the legs through the back of the throat was quite disorganized, and so the work I would do peripherally would be preparation. I might end up doing three 4th hours spread through the series, because that is the primary restriction in the organism. So, if I only did one 4th hour, and I was seeing [what I described], I would not be true to what I was seeing.

"I will often book a Ten Series and tell people that I may have less or more sessions to the point where I think they've reached a state shift so that they can move into the next pattern. I may find that I'm doing several rounds of extremity work because the strains are all jammed up in the extremities. If you can't get the plasticity and the opening up in the arms and legs, nothing in the middle can change. So you're observing these restrictions. For example, you may be looking at a kyphosis or a scoliosis or a collapsed chest, and if you think 'Oh my God, the arms and legs can't accommodate this. If they are not addressed they're going to keep telling the body to go back to its primary pattern,' then I would shift my focus to the extremities more strongly.

"I'm still working with the same goals that are imbedded in Dr. Rolf's series – [the goals] that each session is looking to manifest. I would go down the list and postulate which [goals] are 'in place,' which ones are 'close,' and which ones are 'far away.' In this sense I really changed how I went about [accomplishing those goals], but it is based on Ida's principles and order of development...My own experience then is...that I think the Recipe and the principles that are hidden in it are the foundation of Rolfing, [but] that how you apply it [might vary]. Because if you couldn't go to the person's individual fixations beyond what the Recipe would handle, you couldn't get there [and get the changes you wanted]. So really, around the advanced work was where my big change in Rolfing happened. What drove our political breakdown was this issue. I wanted to figure out what are the principles that make Rolfing operate as opposed to what is the formula that makes it work. [I wanted to] teach the students to work from principle rather than from formula. So in the school that I'm in, we have gone there. We're teaching the work, particularly beyond the basic work, as principle driven rather than formula driven." – *Interview in Espanola, New Mexico, March 14, 2004.*

Tom Wing

Interviewer: Do you still use the Ten-Session Series in your practice for people who are new to Rolfing?

Tom: "Well, yes and no. One thing to remember about Ida is that she was always experimenting with her recipes. It wasn't as much with the basic Ten, although even there she would sometimes throw something in that if you checked with somebody in an earlier class [hadn't been there previously]. It wasn't a complete work. None of her stuff was a complete piece of work, where she just had finished with it. She was always working on what she'd done. It showed up more in the advanced class where she was never happy with the advanced series.

"I remember one time Jan and I were having a discussion about the 4th session; this is when we were doing a five-session advanced series. I said, 'Well the 4th session is this' and he said, 'No it isn't, that's not the 4th session, the 4th session is this.' And he laid it out and I said, 'No it isn't it's this.' He said, 'No it isn't it's this.' I said, 'Well look, I was just in class and I just got it from Ida and it's this.' He said, 'Well I was in class and it was that.' And then we realized, yeah, she used every class as an experiment to try out

I feel like Dr. Rolf gave me my life…she took me out of one world and gave me another world…The Rolfing gives me a paradigm for understanding my experience in this world in a way that I didn't have before. I tend to interpret my world experiences now and view them through the Rolfing lens of what I learned from her. I consider Ida a Teacher in the capital 'T' sense. She was a great Teacher.

– TOM WING

different ways of [accomplishing her goals] to see what would happen in the class. If something didn't work well, [then] she could do something about it. She was always working on it.

"But the Ten was more set. It really was. But I got dissatisfied with what I'd learned in 1973 as the Ten Series in a lot of different ways. At that point what we were passing around clandestinely among ourselves were the recipes that we weren't supposed to do. Ida didn't like it. She said, 'You are not supposed to do that. Watch what I'm doing and [then] listen to what I'm saying and get [a recipe] together for yourself.' But no, we were so insecure that we would [go] out behind the barn and swap recipes. I got mine from Roger out in California. What I did at some point before I started teaching was to redefine the Ten-Session Series for myself and to try to bring it down to what I considered to be the most basic aspects that the sessions had in common in the various recipes."

Interviewer: There was more than one Ten-Session Series Recipe?

Tom: "There were different ones, but the sequence always stayed the same in all the recipes that I saw, although what you did varied."

Interviewer: Did the principles stay the same?

Tom: "…the principles stayed the same, and that's what I tried to do; [I tried] to get it down to the simplest statement of the principles of the session to see if working from that point of view – going back to the principles and deriving my own application and my own way of using them to see – would be useful. [I'd ask myself:] 'Would that satisfy me and would it get the results [I wanted to see]?' I got [the sessions] down to basically a series of areas and interrelationships, and that was it. [For example], the first session is about these [particular] areas and functions and their interrelationships…[I'd ask myself:] 'What interrelationships are being worked with? What are the functions you are working with? And what are the results you desire to see?' It became areas and relationships, then moves and techniques. I find that useful.

"I still find that [approach] useful, and I will diverge from it when it feels right. My first thought [is]: 'Can I apply this? Does this seem like a rational and logical way to progress with this person's process?' If it is, then I follow it. [It is] common sense, like the first session opening the chest, opening the breathing function. Now opening the breathing function might mean that I go somewhere that I never would have gone before and do things I never would have done in 1984, but I still keep that [goal of opening the breathing] in mind. [I ask myself:] 'What is the progression of the functions and does that still hold?'"

Interviewer: You then kept the relationships, the functions, the general principles and goals of that progression of the Ten Series over the years? For example, you first open the breathing, and then you begin on the base of support.

Tom: "Yes and no again. Let me put it this way. The Recipe as I understand it is always in the back of my mind. Ida always intended it as a vehicle to get you into the work and not as something that *was* the work. I really believe that. This was her way of passing on a way to get in and do something that had a logical sequence and a logical expectation for result. But, once you had worked in that area for long enough, then she didn't see that you were going to always do the same thing. That's not what I got from her. She'd talk about chefs and cooks, and recipes [being] for cooks. Once you learn why the recipe is done the way it is…then you learn what you want to do. She said that when you understand those principles and their applications and what's essential and what isn't and how to play with that to get the results you want, then you're a chef, and you go ahead and you don't need the Recipe; it's in there.

"For years and years now my basic study in doing the work has been to listen to the body, what Ida would have called 'seeing the body.'…Ida used to say, 'Well don't just stand there looking, get your hands in there and see what's going on.' I put myself in a place where I am listening to the body. I'm trying to get the information from the person's body as to what needs to happen. What's the first thing? What's the next thing? Where is it going? Then [I would] just *be there* for that information, constantly, while I'm working, rather than having an idea in my head of where we're going. (Although I do have an idea in my head of where we're going, of course.)

"That Recipe [is] imprinted in there…I find that when someone comes in…I'll listen to their body and I'll do…whatever I think should be done, and it may or may not fit into the 'one through ten.' But generally, in retrospect, when I look back on the process I do with people. It tends to [follow the Ten-Series pattern]. I go, 'Well *hmm.* I sort of did do it, didn't I?' I could reinterpret it and say, "Yes, I did the Recipe," or in watching myself I could go "Well no, I didn't do the Recipe, I did something entirely different." – *Interview in Olympia, Washington, March 25, 2004.*

ALICE'S STORY

Alice first came to me after having had the basic Ten Series from another Rolfer. She loved Rolfing and wanted to continue working with her back and neck pain. As a result of an accident, Alice had received some severe whiplash that was manifesting as pain and tightness all down her left side, from neck through to her lower leg. I could see the pattern of twist, particularly in the front part of her neck, in the sternocleidomastoid muscle being pulled to the left and the constriction radiating down the left arm and into her hip. When I began to work on her upper back, the tissue had that familiar feel of whiplash trauma – hard and unyielding. We worked slowly all over her body steadily for about twelve sessions. As the outer compensatory patterns began to release, and the connective tissue and musculature began to become more resilient, I started to see an underlying pattern that was so intricate that I would be hard pressed to describe it. One day, after I had focused quite a few sessions on her legs, hips, and ribcage, I felt it was time to come again directly to her neck and shoulder pattern and work there. She was very quiet in this session and, after I had done some good strong work directly on the hard tissue in her upper back, I worked slowly and meditatively unwinding the twist in her neck and how it related into her head. We got quite a shift, and she said she felt her whole left side was up off the bed, and her eyes were turned to the right. At that point I saw that the release in her neck had revealed a whole intricate pattern of compensation in her ribcage and back, which had been holding in response to the twist in her neck. In that instant I could clearly see the pattern, but wasn't sure

The results of Rolfing are as varied as the people getting Rolfed. From the cellular to the gross physical level something becomes mobile and resilient, which before was held tight and rigid. There is more length and space throughout the body, better integration and organization of the physical structure. Movement is freer and the stance is more upright.

– BETSY SISE

how to unravel it, it was so deep. We were nearing the end of the session and I didn't want to enter a new area, but to integrate her in relationship to the changes she had gotten. So I asked her to get in touch with the bottoms of her feet and move up through hips and all the way up her spine and out the top of her head with her awareness. She is a wonderfully enthusiastic client and was easily able to do this.

As Alice's consciousness would touch on a particular area I could feel the subtle changes under my hands. Then I asked her to get in touch with the whole right side of her body, then with the whole left side. The minute she shifted her awareness to her left side her whole body dropped back on the left and little minute shifts and adjustments were happening right and left. We were both observing in amazement the wisdom of the body in action. She was able to just "be there" with it and allow it to happen.

Her eyes felt better, but they still felt a bit shifted to the right. After the integrative pelvic lift, I had her sit up. Then I rested my hands lightly on top of her head to feel the relationship of her spine to her eyes. In my experience, the eyes organize around the spine to give a sense of kinesthetic center around any spinal aberration, so when there is a change in the alignment of the spine, the eyes need to adjust to create a new kinesthetic center.

As she sat there, with her feet grounded on the floor, I asked her to keep her eyes open and to slowly turn to the right, leading with her eyes and going no faster than she could let her spine and body respond to the turn. I monitored this from my light contact with the top of her head where I could feel if she was turning as a whole, or needed to tune in to a specific spot. We repeated this to the left, and then she was able to naturally find the new kinesthetic sense of center. When she stood up we were both amazed at the deep change that had taken place. I pointed out to her that her own inner wisdom had really made the change, and I had just helped her to access it.

Alice speaks here about her decision to get Rolfed and her experience of Rolfing.

It was 1973. "Benjamin" was one of several staff associated with the facility where I was employed. Everyone experienced Benjamin as a very quiet, reserved individual, whose posture and demeanor portrayed him as not very confident and rather tentative. He spoke very softly and avoided eye contact, which was aided by his long hair that shielded most of his face. Although he was tall, over six feet, he seemed shorter because of his hunched shoulders and bowed head.

Our work schedules varied such that I didn't see Benjamin on a regular basis. However, I recall most vividly seeing him after some period of time. I hardly recognized him. He stood tall, shoulders back, with direct eye contact, confident voice and demeanor, and with neatly groomed hair that framed his fully visible face. Something had transformed him. Everyone was amazed at the dramatic change. He announced that it was all the result of Rolfing. At that moment, I knew with total certainty that someday, at the right opportunity, I too would experience the transforming effects of Rolfing.

The power of love to change bodies is legendary, built into folklore, common sense, and everyday experience. Love moves the flesh, it pushes matter around... Throughout history, "tender loving care" has uniformly been recognized as a valuable element in healing.

– Larry Dossey

Several years passed. Many experiences occurred. From time to time, I casually heard about, and was vaguely interested in, various approaches to bodywork and the results to be expected. It wasn't until I had experienced an accumulation of physical discomforts and sought numerous avenues of relief that the concept of Rolfing was once again presented to me. Just as I had declared several years earlier, the right opportunity arrived for me to experience the transforming effects of Rolfing.

Like most people who decide to avail themselves of Rolfing, I had specific physical discomforts and I was anticipating relief. My most capable and sensitive massage therapist had suggested that I consider Rolfing to address the more chronic conditions for which her massage could provide only temporary respite. So it was from the perspective of relieving specific physical discomforts that I embarked upon a series of Rolfing sessions. Relief of those specific physical discomforts was definitely realized over the course of the initial sessions. However, something else, totally unanticipated, also was experienced.

Although not as dramatic and obvious as the transformation I had seen years earlier in my colleague, as my Rolfing sessions progressed I began to experience not only a physical, but also an emotional, mental and spiritual transformation. This transformation was at times immediate and specific. At other times, it was very general and subtle. Either way, the transformation was always experienced as a major "Wow, that's amazing and so powerful!"

The initial Rolfing sessions brought relief from what I later defined as the surface, more gross, physical discomforts. As these more gross physical discomforts began to dissolve, other more subtle physical discomforts seemed to emerge from deeper levels. As the deeper levels began to dissolve, I began to realize that the physical discomforts were mirror images, or physical counterparts to my emotional, mental and spiritual discomforts. With each resolution of a physical discomfort, I experienced the resolution of some deeper discomfort that resided within my inner self. I began to experience in very direct ways how my physical body is a reflection of my emotional, mental and spiritual bodies.

The relationship between my physical body and my inner self was most directly realized through significant changes in my breath and breathing. Each resolution of a physical discomfort was specifically connected to changes in my ability to breathe more deeply, more fully, and more completely. I intuitively realized that more breath meant more energy to my blood cells, more vitality to my nerves, and more life to my organs and all my body's interrelated functions. I began to realize the Eastern wisdom that teaches the vital role of breath in creating and sustaining Life.

As I was able to breathe more deeply and completely, I began to experience a transformation of my inner self. Lifelong limiting thoughts, beliefs and attitudes about myself seemed to dissipate and dissolve, liberating me to a more positive and healthier

Finally there is the light breath, *which is what I call the breath that feeds the soul. This energy is part of the spiritual force of the universal energy, and it enters your body with every breath.*
– ROBERT C. FULFORD, D.O., *DR. FULFORD'S TOUCH OF LIFE*, 40.

perspective. I realized how my fears and insecurities had restricted my breath in both direct and subtle ways and that, in turn, my restricted breath had manifested in my physical, emotional, mental and spiritual discomforts.

My Rolfing experiences enabled me to realize that my physical body is a mirror of my inner sense of self. As my body began to experience realignment with its physical structure, my emotional, mental and spiritual self began to come into alignment. Restructuring my physical body allowed the restructuring of my emotional, mental and spiritual bodies. The effects of this process were reciprocal and cumulative. The more my physical body experienced alignment, the more I experienced an alignment of my inner self. The more my inner self became aligned, the more my physical body expressed its natural alignment.

I discovered that realignment of my physical body resolved physical discomforts. In so doing, it also liberated my breath, dissipated fears and insecurities, and produced a reintegration of my inner self for a greater sense of well being and vitality. For me Rolfing is method of experiencing and sustaining a more meaningful and enjoyable life.

Endnotes, Chapter 5

[1] Robert Schleip, "Primary Reflexes and Structural Typology." *Rolf Lines*. October, 1993.
[2] Rolf class notes from Peter Melchior.
[3] Rolf class notes. Tom Wing.

[4] Rolf class notes.

[5] Rolf class notes. Tom Wing.

[6] Rolf class notes.

[7] Melchior, Peter. Interview. Lyons, Colorado. March 4, 2004.

[8] Rolf, Ida P. Ph.D. *Rolfing: The Integration of Human Structures*. Santa Monica, California: Dennis-Landman, 1977, 112.

[9] Hamilton, W.J. Ed. *Textbook of Human Anatomy: Second Edition*. Saint Louis, Missouri: The C.V. Mosby Company, 1976, 181.

[10] Ibid., 664.

[11] Rolf class notes. Emmett Hutchins.

[12] Ibid.

[13] Clemente, Carmine, Ph.D. *Anatomy: A Regional Atlas of the Human Body*. Philadelphia, Pennsylvania: Lea and Febiger, 1975. Figures 377 -380.

[14] Rolf class notes, Jan Sultan.

[15] Jeff Linn interview. Boulder, Colorado. March 5, 2004.

[16] Hamilton, W.J. Ed. *Textbook of Human Anatomy*, Second Edition. Saint Louis, Missouri: The CV Mosby Company, 1976, 51.

[17] Rolf class notes, Emmett Hutchins.

[18] Feitis, Rosemary. Editor. *Ida Rolf Talks About Rolfing and Physical Reality*. New York, N.Y.: Harper and Row, 1978, 188.

Part III
The Experience

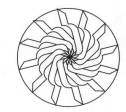

6

What Happens When You Get Rolfed?

The Body/Mind – Overview

I am sitting here in a body that is apparently separate from my surroundings. I am aware of my breath and heartbeat. If I really focus, I might even be aware of the blood coursing through my blood vessels. My awareness is more clearly focused on the feeling of the muscles in my arm and hand as I write, my bare feet on the carpet, my legs and pelvis against the chair. I am not aware of digestive juices or hormones being formed to travel throughout my body. I am not aware of tiny molecules called peptides that are carrying information back and forth from the major systems of my body. Though I can feel my heart beat, I am not aware that my heart creates an electromagnetic field that interacts with the electromagnetic fields of other organs in my body.

I am aware of the air around me, the immediate space in my house, my present mood. I seem to be separate from my surroundings, yet on closer examination I am clearly interacting with what I consider "inner," my body's functions, and "outer," – which I see around me in the environment. When I look at a shadow cast by a tree in the sun, it appears that there is a clear demarcation between the shadow and the sun. But if I look more closely, the demarcation between light and dark becomes less clear, until I can't find the line where light ends and the shadow begins. Thus I am both microcosm and macrocosm, living within and surrounding myriads of microcosms and macrocosms, and there is no clear demarcation, only communication.

The hands, presence, and intention of the Rolfer (or anyone for that matter) enter into this field we call a body-mind, which interacts with a larger field called the gravitational field. Asking the question of this chapter "What happens when you get Rolfed?" will not yield a definitive answer, but will be a stab at an ongoing process.

Once, as a teenager, I listened to my father and a bunch of MIT professors and scientists talking, of all things, about the merits or demerits of prefrontal lobotomy. Suddenly I had this odd thought, that all the guys with the microscopes looking for smaller and smaller things, and all the guys with the telescopes looking for bigger and bigger things further and further away, would eventually come full circle until they were looking at each other. Perhaps we have always been looking at each other but not really seeing. In some situations, photos of planets and galaxies can look remarkably similar to photos of atoms and molecules if one looks at them as fields of energy, as Dr. Rolf did in describing simple salt crystals:

Thus an organic substance, salt, originally thought of as a molecule consisting of a union between two atoms, can be more precisely evaluated if the atoms are seen as energy fields, patterned solar systems whirling in balanced orbits.[1]

Back in the 1960s and 1970s Dr. Rolf was asking questions about the relationship of the energy field of the human being with the gravitational field of the earth.

We are simultaneously matter and spirit. In order to understand ourselves and be healthy in both body and spirit, we have to understand how matter and spirit interact, what draws the spirit or life force out of our bodies, and how we can retrieve our spirits from the false gods of fear, anger, and attachments to the past.

– CAROLINE MYSS, PH.D., *ANATOMY OF THE SPIRIT*, 77.

Nobody can prove what I am about to say, but I think it is so: every energy in which we live is nourishment to us. It is something which is literally contributing food to the individual. If you are living in a field of light, your eyes probably are good; as you deprive yourself of light consistently, the eyes starve and eventually you can't see...Now it would be absolutely ridiculous if we lived in a field of gravity and it had no effect on us, yet down through the ages this has been our assumption, that it didn't make any difference.[2]

In his book *The Biology of Transcendence*, Joseph Chilton Pearce wrote: "As with most forces, we know fields not as themselves alone but through the results of their function or actions. No man has seen gravity, but we assume there is a force we call gravity because things fall to center."[3] Dr. Rolf was postulating that the field of gravity interacts with structure by noticing how the body functioned when better aligned.

In 1998, Mae Wan Ho, a brilliant scientist, published a book called *The Rainbow and the Worm: The Physics of Organisms*. In it she describes a remarkable discovery; organisms are actually liquid crystalline structures:

What is the liquid crystalline state? It is a state or phase of matter in between the solid and the liquid. Unlike liquids that have little or no molecular order, liquid crystals have an orientational order, in that the molecules are aligned in some common directions, rather like a crystal. But unlike solid crystals, liquid crystals are flexible, malleable, and responsive.[4]

Even though Ho doesn't specifically mention gravity, it is remarkable that this scientific discovery of the 1990s so reflects, on the molecular level, Dr. Rolf's interest in alignment, and her belief that the spatial arrangement of a substance would ultimately change its behavior. Regarding a salt crystal she states:

> …arrangement in space is fundamental to the behavior of a substance, however simple it may be…microscopic examination shows crystals whose edges are sharply defined and whose plane surfaces meet at specific and definite angles. Any deviation from these indices indicates an admixture of some other material, a so-called "impurity." Significantly, any deviation makes the chemical behavior less predictable.[5]

As the internal and external environments of the physical body are in constant interaction, so are the so-called "mind" and body. In her paper *Gravity: An Unexplored Factor in the More Human Use of Human Beings*, Dr. Rolf asks:

> What is an integrated man? To the medical specialist, this body, and this alone, IS the man. To the psychiatrist the body is less than the man; it is merely the externalized expression of personality. Neither of these specialists has accepted as real a third possibility; namely that in some way, as yet poorly defined, the physical body is actually the personality, rather than its expression; is the energy unit we call man, as it exists in its material 3-dimensional reality.[6]

The hypothesis that the physical body actually is the personality is taken up later by the work of Dr. Candace Pert, Ph.D., which she reports in her book *The Molecules of Emotion: Why You Feel The Way You Feel*. Dr. Pert is a neuroscientist who in 1972 discovered the opiate receptor. She continued with pioneering research on how the chemicals in our body form an information network linking mind and body. In her studies she found that, at the molecular level, there is really no distinction between mind and body. She describes this interaction between mind and body as follows:

> We are now ready to explore my theory that these bio-chemicals [neuropeptides] are the physiological substrates of emotion, the molecular underpinnings of what we experience as feelings, sensations, thoughts, drives, perhaps even spirit and soul.[7]…The body is the unconscious mind! Repressed traumas caused by overwhelming emotion can be stored in a body part, thereafter affecting our ability to feel that part or even move it.[8]

Dr. Pert uses the word "emotions" to describe states such as anger, fear, sadness, while Dr. Rolf uses the broader term "personality." Dr. Pert, Dr. Mae Wan Ho and Dr. Rolf were powerful and creative women. Each in her own way and time was examining similar ideas about the nature of the interactions among mind, body and environment. I would love to have gathered them together in a room and listened in. I think Dr. Rolf would have greatly appreciated hearing of the discoveries of Ho and Pert, which supported her ideas – ideas that predated the tools that are available today to measure and observe things like peptides and the liquid crystalline structure of the body.

I had often wondered about the chemical interactions between the body and emotions. In graduate school in 1967, I came to a state of near nervous breakdown. I finally went to a doctor who found out that I was anemic. After taking iron tablets for a while I felt totally different – no longer controlled by the extreme emotions that had plagued me before. I remember questioning at the time whether I was just a bunch of chemicals, given that one chemical change affected my whole disposition. As these three

To exist as separate beings, to be manifest on the material plane as we are, we must be both a part of the fabric of nature and independent of it. This dual requirement determines two basic energy flows in our bodies: one conducts energy through the body and connects us with nature; the other relates to the circulation of energy within the body and organizes us as individuals.

– FRITZ FREDERICK SMITH, M.D., INNER BRIDGES, 27.

women scientists have said, each in her own way, the body and the mind, feelings and physiology are at some level inseparable.

Dr. Rolf intuitively knew – from her background in biochemistry, her studies of osteopathy and homeopathy, as well as her own deep spiritual and metaphysical nature – that to make a change in one area of the body would result in change throughout. She chose to work with the connective-tissue system directly, with her hands. She chose the system that is the organ of communication and form.

As we continue to look at what happens when you get Rolfed, keep in mind that life is a process involving ongoing communication. When I get Rolfed I feel many things going on at once, such as the pressure of the Rolfer's hands, the stretching and releasing of the connective tissue, the places where I am holding, the movement of my breath and the content of my thoughts. But there are deeper levels of change of which I may not be aware. There are changes that continue in waves of unseen and unfelt interactions deep within my body, and these changes may only manifest months later, and in ways that I may not even connect with the fact of having been Rolfed.

The Physiological Aspect of the Body-Mind

The Connective Tissue System

When I recognize a friend walking toward me in the distance, I see a specific form within the general form of the human being. Yes, that's Annie's walk, the rhythm with which she moves, the way she swings her arms. The way those legs are shaped are Annie's; her erect spine, her size, weight, height and the way the flesh is distributed on her skeletal frame make up the familiar form. What I see in a general sense is the large connective-tissue system – of bones, tendons, ligaments, fascia, cartilage...– that make up the form of the body.

The fascia, the thinnest and most changeable of these tissues, is a thin elastic three-dimensional web that exists everywhere in the body. Fascia envelops every structure – from bones and muscles all the way to the cellular level. Fascia consists of an extracellular matrix of collagen, elastin, and groundsubstance that surrounds all cells, skin, bones, cartilage, tendons, walls of the arteries and veins, alimentary canal, air passages, and membranes covering all organs.[9] According to Dr. Ho: "Actually *all* the cells in the body are in turn interconnected to one another via connective tissues as has been pointed out by biochemist James Oschman nearly fifteen years ago. It is responsible for the form and posture we see in each person."[10]

Louis Schultz, Ph.D. and Rosemary Feitis, D.O. have called the fascia "the endless web," in their book titled *The Endless Web: Fascial Anatomy and Physical Reality.*

I have often thought about webs in considering the web of the spider. There are certain appropriate patterns of relational tension that hold the web in its intended form. When a fly lands in the web, then the tensional pattern changes and the spider can feel it and know where the fly is. But the human fascial web is a three-dimensional sphere as Dr. Rolf points out:

> The body is a web of fascia. A spider web is in a plane; this web is in a sphere. We can trace the lines of that web to get an understanding of how what we see in a body works. For example, why, when we work with the superficial fascia, does this change the tone of the fascia as a whole?[11]

When I am Rolfing I can often feel "where the fly has landed." It might be a point of impact from a fall. When I apply some

I stand in awe of my body.

– HENRY DAVID
THOREAU

I had two skiing injuries, one to my left ankle and one to my left knee. I remember the session on my feet and legs from Ed Taylor, my first Rolfer. Afterward I went walking in the desert in my sandals and the first thing I noticed was that I wasn't kicking sand into the sandal from scooping outward with my left foot. I could feel the action of my arches and toes. It wasn't just one big block of unconsciousness from the knees down, but an alive feeling. There were individual muscles there!
— BETSY SISE

pressure to the fascia with my hands, I can feel the tensional pattern throughout this web of connective tissue. Clients also will often feel a release in an area of the body quite removed from where I am working. Strains in one place in the system will affect the web everywhere. As a simple example, sit relatively straight in a chair. Straighten out your shirt so it is even and smooth on the front. Now pull the lower left-hand corner of your shirt down and slightly to the left and notice the patterns of strain in the rest of the shirt, especially in the right clavicle and shoulder area. Now imagine that this pattern has been locked into your structure for years. If your right shoulder begins to hurt and loses mobility, it would be tempting to work there first because that is where you feel the pain. But we must consider the whole – there is a pattern of imbalance that needs to be attended to.

"Lift" is another aspect to consider in the structure of connective tissue as a system. Dr. Rolf insisted that when a body was properly aligned and integrated, gravity would lift the body up, as Emmett Hutchins mentioned when talking about his experience of moving toward weightlessness (*see* Chapter 4). The soft tissue should support the weight, not the bones. "The spine is not a column. A column supports weight from the top. The spine is an up-ended beam and should be posterior."[12] How can gravity, which pulls something down, lift something up? We must look at this seeming paradox from a different angle. Instead of looking at the body as a compression model with columns supporting weight from above, we can look at it as a system of tensegrity masts. The term "tensegrity" or "tensional integrity" was first developed in 1948 by Buckminster Fuller as an architectural principle often seen in tents and geodesic domes. According to Oschman :

A tensegrity system is characterized by a continuous tensional network (tendons) connected by a discontinuous set of compressive elements (struts). A tensegrity structure

forms a stable yet dynamic system that interacts efficiently and resiliently with forces acting upon it.[13]

Ron Kirkby, Ph.D., an early Rolfer, wrote a fascinating article
called "The Probable Reality Behind Structural Integration: How
Gravity Supports the Body." He puts forth the hypothesis that the
theory of tensegrity could give some clues to what Dr. Rolf meant
when she said, "Gravity lifts the body up." Most of what we see
around us in buildings, for instance, is columnar structures bearing
compressive loads. Kirkby uses a balloon to demonstrate a tensional structure that is able to bear weight. He suggests that you
partially inflate a balloon, put it on a table, and then balance a ball
on top of the balloon. As the balloon is partially inflated, the
weight of the ball forms a cup in the balloon and the ball is supported there.[14] Describing the basic idea in a tensegrity structure,
Kirkby writes:

> The whole structure can stand on its own because it rep-
> resents a series of vector equilibria, a vector being a force
> with a specific direction, and "equilibrium" meaning that
> the forces balance exactly so that they cancel each other
> out…The whole structure is stable because every force is
> balanced by an opposing force.[15]
>
> In sum, too great a tension anywhere in the structure
> causes shortening and rotations, though not necessarily in
> the area of too-great tension. Correcting bends and rota-
> tions, then, consists in easing off local tensions, so that the
> structure can assume its proper length and unwind its rota-
> tions. (Sound familiar?)[16]

Yes, it sounds familiar to a Rolfer because this is exactly where
we begin – easing off tension and bringing length and space into
the body. The sense of lift and lightness often felt directly after a

Rolfing session is the result of the tensional forces in the web of connective tissue being balanced. The bones then become more like bracers or struts rather than weight bearing columns. Kirkby then presents an interesting yet obvious idea that it is gravity that sets these tensions in the human body, noting that: "Muscles act as units because the fascia of each little muscle cell is interwoven with the fascia of all the rest. When gravity pulls on the muscle, then, it sets an even tension throughout the muscle and through it into the planes of fascia of which the muscle is a part."[17]

We have seen the effects on astronauts of being out of the gravity field. For starters, muscles weaken and the body shortens. I once had a similar experience of this shortening when spending some time in one of John Lilly's sensory deprivation tanks. The tank, somewhat like a coffin only a little more spacious (not much!), is filled with warm salt water. It is thickly insulated against sound. I would get in, close the lid, and float in the salt water. While my mind and emotions went through some strong reactions, I could feel my body shortening into my habitual structural patterns, and I did not get the feeling of lift through the spine that I do when sitting in meditation or standing in the normal gravity field. Someday, perhaps, a Rolfer will do some studies with astronauts on the effects on the body of being out of the gravitational field.

Kirkby concludes:

I offer the following hypothesis: when a human being has all his different segments lined up along a vertical line, then the tensions in the tensional networks of the body, the fascia are set to such a level by *gravity*, that the structure stands up by itself, and reaches its maximum extension. A shorter way of saying this is to say that gravity supports the body by setting the correct tensions within the upright man. An even shorter way of saying this is to say that gravity supports the body, lifts it up.[18]

In terms of what might be happening when you get Rolfed, we are looking at how the strain in one area of a coherent system affects the whole body. This is why Rolfers are first lengthening and thus decompressing areas of the fascia. When there is more length and space, compressions, amazingly enough, release upwards, and thus the feeling of lightness and lift.

To venture deeper into the cellular structure of connective tissue we find that "…the entire cell is mechanically and electrically interconnected in a 'solid state' or 'tensegrity system.'"[19] Dr. Mae Wan Ho explains further:

> The entire cell acts as a coherent whole, so information or disturbance to one part propagates promptly to all other parts. Biomechanist and cell biologist Donald Ingber proposed the idea that the whole cell and its "solid state" of membrane, skeleton, cytoskeleton, microtrabecular lattice and nuclear scaffold, form an interconnected "tensegrity system" that always deforms or changes *as a whole* when local stresses and strains are experienced.[20]

I find this a remarkable discovery. Not only is the general connective-tissue system arranged in balanced tensional relationships, but even at the cellular level the same system of tensegrity applies. For those interested in further details on cellular biology and physics, both Mae Wan Ho's book (*The Rainbow and the Worm: The Physics of Organisms*) and that of James Oschman (*Energy Medicine: The Scientific Basis*) contain well-researched reports of science that corroborates this deep intercommunication and constant distribution of information everywhere throughout the body-mind continuum.

As a Rolfer, when I use my hands to contact this connective tissue system of tensegrity masts with the intention of creating length and space, I envision little releases of compression, twists,

[T]he human body is surrounded by something that I call a life field…[which] conveys vitality to your physical body and provides you with your spirit. Whenever you feel a disturbance or an injury, the life field manifests its shock in the physical body with a depletion of energy. If left unchecked, this deficiency can lead to dysfunction, disease, and, ultimately, to the body's total collapse; but if the deficiency is discovered and restored, the body can repair the health that it has lost…

— ROBERT FULFORD, D.O.

and snags in the body-stocking of fascia. I, and often the client too, can feel wavelike releases that radiate from where I have the contact. This touch, and the awareness of the client are communicating information all the way to the cellular level and beyond. This amazing recognition is rather humbling, I'd say, yet filled with possibility.

* * *

From our brief look at connective tissue and cells as tensegrity systems we can see how establishing length and space, and then working for order in the body's relationship to gravity, can bring great relief to many chronic structural problems. To see the body as an integral set of finely-tuned tensional forces that are actually coming into balance when in relation to gravity, gives an idea of why Dr. Rolf might make the statement, "Gravity is the therapist." By thinking and seeing in terms of relationships rather than cause and effect, we trust that given the proper chance, as the body comes into alignment, gravity will act in a positive way. Emmett Hutchins put it well when he said, "Primarily I think it [Rolfing] works because that's the way the structure would like to be anyway."[21] The body's natural inclination is to be balanced and aligned in the gravitational field.

The Respiratory System

To continue on our journey of what might be happening when you get Rolfed, let's look at breathing. How might Rolfing affect breathing?

First of all, the fascia and muscles around the ribcage need to be resilient and flexible enough to allow for full rib excursion and thus a full breath. Breath feeds the nervous system with oxygen that is carried by the blood. Breath is literally life – we don't live longer than a few minutes without breathing. Breath is governed by the autonomic nervous system, yet we can also consciously control our breathing, giving us the inherent power to influence our own body chemistry. The practice of *pranayama* in the yogic tradition is one example of this. Another more common method of controlled breathing is practiced by women giving birth. Such breathing will lessen pain and allow the body to do its natural job. Dr. Candace Pert briefly describes the role of breathing and how the body's own opiates – endorphins – are found in the respiratory system.

> Conscious breathing, the technique employed by both the yogi and the woman in labor, is extremely powerful. There is a wealth of data showing that changes in the rate and depth of breathing produce changes in the quantity and kind of peptides that are released from the brain stem…By bringing this process into consciousness and doing something to alter it – either holding your breath or breathing extra fast – you cause the peptides to diffuse rapidly throughout the cerebrospinal fluid, in an attempt to restore homeostasis, the body's feedback mechanism for restoring and maintaining balance…Virtually any peptide found anywhere else can be found in the respiratory center. This peptide substrate may provide the scientific rationale for the powerful healing effects of consciously controlled breath patterns.[22]

I've got to keep breathing. It'll be my worst business mistake if I don't.

– STEVE MARTIN

The feeling of a truly *open* breath is virtually unbeatable, as I have felt the ecstasy of it a few times in meditation. Tom Wing and Jan Sultan both noted (*see* Chapter 1, on Dr. Rolf) the opening of the breath as being the key thing that caught their attention about Rolfing. In any kind of emotional or physical trauma, breathing is affected. I will often have clients who are so restricted in their breathing that I wonder how they are even walking

Our thoughts, regardless of their content, first enter our systems as energy. Those that carry emotional, mental, psychological, or spiritual energy produce biological responses that are then stored in our cellular memory. In this way our biographies are woven into our biological systems, gradually, slowly, every day.

– CAROLINE MYSS, PH.D., *ANATOMY OF THE SPIRIT*, 40.

around, yet they are functioning "normally." When I ask them to take a breath and observe what they do, I am sometimes incredulous, "Was that it? Did I miss something?" I think to myself. "I hardly saw the ribs move at all." I understand the phenomenon, however, as I have felt this restriction many times in my own body. When I am emotionally upset or stressed out the first thing that starts to shut down is my breathing. When I used to ski race in downhill competition the coach taught us to breathe by making a whistling noise through the teeth so that we could hear ourselves and remember to breathe. As I have no depth perception due to an eye injury as a child, a downhill ski race was about two minutes of sheer terror. To this day, whenever I am in a stressful situation and must take action, I use that method of breathing taught to me by that ski coach.

To put it simply, breath is the life force that flows through the body. When breathing is jammed due to trauma, often beginning at birth, oxygen intake is restricted and there just isn't as much energy flowing through the body. For this reason, breathing is one of the first things that is addressed in the first hour of Rolfing, as Dr. Rolf states:

> When the position of the ribs is changed, breathing changes…Now there isn't anyone that knows so little about biological chemistry that he doesn't understand that getting more air into the lungs and getting it moving faster is going to change the chemistry of every cell in the body. So in a first Rolfing hour, we have started changing the chemistry of every cell in the body in the first ten minutes…All of a sudden the skin becomes pink; the skin may be a little more moist – the glands of the skin are working.[23]

As noted in Chapter 5, *The Basic Ten-Session Series*, not only breathing itself, but breathing through the nose, as opposed to mouth breathing, is vital to good health. Dr. Robert Fulford, a talented cranial osteopath, stated this directly:

> Remember: always try to breathe through your nostrils and not your mouth, because air must contact the olfactory nerves to stimulate your brain and put it into its natural rhythm. If you don't breathe through your nose, in a sense you are only half alive.[24]

In my experience Fulford's words are so true. On the rare occasion when I have a cold and can't breathe through my nose I do feel half alive! This is why as Rolfers we have a technique for working inside the nose. As strange as this procedure sounds, it has provided many, myself included, with great relief by allowing me to breathe more freely through the nose.

The work of Dr. Sutherland, an osteopath who developed cranial osteopathy, had a deep influence on Dr. Rolf, as she states here from *Ida Rolf Talks*:

> What Dr. Sutherland was teaching, and what seemingly did come from the great mystic and scientist Swedenborg, was not merely that there were reflex points on the head, but that the head was part of the respiratory system. He taught that respiration was not a movement of the lungs, except secondarily; it was a movement of the head, which by this movement pumped spinal fluid through the spinal column…This idea of respiration as a basic function of the nervous system is a revolutionary idea. Breathing thus represents the functional communication between…myofascial and neural tissue…Respiration is accompanied by movement in the sacrum…This acts as a pump for cerebrospinal fluid…It acts as a pump for the entire spinal

mechanism...presumably, to the brain, which is part of the spinal mechanism.[25]

Dr. Rolf sat in on some of Sutherland's classes and brought some of the early ideas of cranial osteopathy into her Rolfing, including the fact that the cranium, sacrum and spine were part of the respiratory system. She saw and felt the breath as movement throughout the body and challenged us to see and feel that even the arches of the feet showed subtle movement in response to breathing. As Rolfers, anywhere in the body that we touch can and will have some effect on the breathing of the client.

When you get Rolfed, not only does your physical pattern of breathing, with all its chemical interactions in the body, change, but you become aware of how you are breathing and thus are able to change old unconsciously held patterns.

Digestion and Elimination

In the most optimal balance of the body, each of the organs in the abdominal area has a specific spatial orientation and location, as well as a subtle pattern of movement. Abdominal muscles that are overly tight, short, and habitually held in rigid patterns confine the digestive and eliminative organs to restricted space and thus limit their proper function. Conversely, abdominal muscles that are flaccid and without tone provide no support for these same organs to maintain their optimal spatial orientation. An anteriorly rotated pelvis leaves the abdominal contents protruding and unsupported. Dr. Rolf noted:

> The facts of physiological function support the assumption that structure determines function. In the musculoskeletal system, function is movement; in the cardiovascular system, it is circulation; in the intricate gut, digestion. All of these systems are imbedded in the myofascial component,

The basic fuel of the body is glucose, or blood sugar, which is the brain's only food. Burning a sugar cube over a gas flame yields a flash of light and heat and a greasy lump of carbon, but the same sugar burned in the brain produces all the thoughts and emotions we have. The Sistine Chapel, Paradise Lost, and Beethoven's Ninth are all accomplishments of burning sugar; so is this book and your ability to read it.

– Deepak Chopra M.D., Ageless Body Timeless Mind, 135

and physiologic activity in any one of them is directly related to spatial balance.[26]

The autonomic nervous system controls all the so-called unconscious aspects of the body such as breathing, digestion, elimination and heart rate. One of the largest plexi of the autonomic nervous system is the lumbar plexus, which lies imbedded in the psoas muscle. Dr. Rolf often mentioned the importance of the psoas muscle and its balance with the rectus abdominus muscle. A properly functioning psoas should lift and support the lumbar vertebrae back. If the psoas, which contains the lumbar plexus imbedded in its fibers, is shortened, rigid, pulled forward, etc., the lumbar plexus will be affected as Dr. Rolf states:

> Structural weakness or metabolic insufficiency in the psoas thereby inevitably affects the lumbar plexus and its autonomic neighbors. If the psoas is inadequate, local nutritional exchange is disturbed, as is the metabolic rate in the lower digestive tract (specifically basic elimination as well as food absorption).[27]

> If the recti, through hyper- or hypotonicity, interfere with the optimal spatial position of the psoas, this reflects into the lumbar plexus and autonomic ganglia, affecting nutrition and tone of the abdominal muscles and viscera.[28]

Will you notice any of this when you get Rolfed? Maybe, and maybe much of it will be below consciousness. When I receive a Rolfing session that addresses my abdominal muscles and psoas I usually feel a great sense of relaxation and peace. Sometimes I will take a huge and refreshing shit (after the session of course!). I often feel my guts growling in a pleasant feeling of release. Most of all, if I have been feeling a bit of low back pain, I feel relief and a

I consider the solar plexus more than just a mass of nerves. I think it is something of an abdominal brain, where the emotions are centered, and from where they are generated. When people say they have a gut feeling, they are literally correct — the feeling does come from the gut. And this is why so many people, when feeling overwhelmed by their emotions, suffer digestive problems.

– ROBERT C. FULFORD, D.O., DR. FULFORD'S TOUCH OF LIFE, 135.

sense of support for my low back along with a feeling of more lift up through my torso. My normally overactive sympathetic nervous system (my flight or fight mechanism) feels calmed down as the parasympathetic nervous system becomes more dominant. So, much of what I feel is more superficial and immediate. The deeper changes may merge into my general life in such a way that I do not necessarily think to attribute later deep changes with having been Rolfed.

As with breathing, the mostly unconscious functions of digestion and elimination can also be brought to conscious awareness, as has been shown with biofeedback methods. Dr. Pert, in working with neuropeptides and their receptors, has found that the mind is as much in the body as it is in the brain itself. The "information molecules" or neuropeptitdes referred to by Pert are found in the lining of the digestive system from the esophagus to the large intestine. Thus, a shift in the connective tissue matrix that supports the organs of digestion and elimination will obviously enhance their function. The connection between the conscious and unconscious aspects of these systems is found in the peptides – or information molecules – that are distributed throughout the autonomic chain of ganglia that run down both sides of the anterior spine.[29] "It is these peptides and their receptors that make the dialog between conscious and unconscious processes possible."[30]

What is this dialog that Candace Pert is pointing to? Let's take it to a strictly muscular level. For example: If you take an object like a tennis ball and grip it tightly in your hand, after a while your hand will start to hurt. But, imagine that you have no idea that you are holding this ball, and you wonder why your hand is hurting. Perhaps you might have been holding this tennis ball unconsciously for a long time without realizing it. Now your hand hurts more and more, but you are still in the dark about why. Somehow you show up in the office of a Rolfer (Smart move!) and she works a bit to open the muscles around your chest so you can breathe a bit better. Then she works a little to release some of the muscles that are locked in your forearm and hand. Your grip loosens and you can begin to feel, *lo and behold*, that you are holding a tennis ball! The Rolfer has you tighten your grip so you can feel yourself engage the muscles of the hand and arm. Then you begin to become conscious of these muscles, as well as the feeling of clenching and letting go. Eventually you experience and become conscious of the muscles that are holding the tennis ball and you consciously let it go. (At last! Thank heavens.)

This is a small and simple example of the dialogue between Rolfer and client, and between the client and her/his own body. A similar dialog is also going on at the cellular and molecular levels. As the Rolfer, when my system begins to enter your fascial system as the client – through my touch, intention and presence – this dialog begins and continues on both the conscious and unconscious levels within us both.

Joints, Muscles, Bones

In the Rolfing paradigm we are considering that bones should act more like spacers rather than weight bearing structures. Joints should work freely without undue restriction, yet they should also work in relation to the central organizing principle of something built around a vertical line of intention. Muscles act in pairs around a joint. Dr. Rolf would say, "When the flexors flex, the extensors should extend." This makes for a more balanced, less stressed joint as well as bones that act more like struts and spacers. The bony vertebrae of the spine protect a key nerve component, a huge network of communication – the spinal cord, nerve roots, and the autonomic chain of ganglia that run down the two sides of the front of the vertebral bodies. Such a communications center should be alive and mobile, thus the spine is not considered a column bearing weight from above. Instead, as Dr. Rolf describes, "In a body reaching toward equipoise, the spine distributes weight

Bones. Two hundred and eight of them. A whole glory turned and tooled. Lo the timbered femur all hung and strapped with beef, whose globate head nuzzles the concave underpart of the pelvis; the little carpals of the wrist faceted as jewels and as jewels named – capitate, lunate, hamate, pisiform; the phalanges, tiny kickshaws of the body, toys fantastic, worn upon the hands and feet like fans of unimagined cleverness; the porcelain pile of the vertebrae atop which rides the domed palanquin of the very brain.

– RICHARD SELZER,
MORTAL LESSONS, 51.

through balance rather than supports it. Here the myofascial structure becomes the key. The bony spine establishes and maintains span in myofascia."[31]

As Rolfers, muscles and fascia are what we directly put our hands on to elicit change. By stretching and reorienting muscles and fascia in space, bones and joints are deeply affected. Fascia is the quickest to change, bones the slowest, but bones do change. I have seen an x-ray of a client with scoliosis both before and after Rolfing and I could see a definite lessening of the scoliosis in the second x-ray. At the time I was quite amazed to actually see that changes could happen at the level of bone.

From the Rolfing standpoint the hip joint – the place where the pelvis meets the leg – is a key joint. The hip joint has far more options for movement than, for example, the surrounding joints of sacroiliac, pubic symphysis, or lumbosacral joints. On the hip joint rests the possibility of the pelvis becoming horizontal. In a horizontal pelvis the anterior superior spines of the iliac crests should be horizontal, thus making the ischial tuberosities level. "Any deviation from the horizontal by the ischial tuberosities always involves a rotation."[32] The vertebral bodies of the spine are able to rotate and if a fixed pattern of rotation happens, the hip joints must compensate. Here is where common low back pain enters the picture.

> …rotations occur as a twisting of the pelvis itself (or the sacrum, 5th lumbar, etc.) around a lower lumbar vertebra. The muscular strain enters awareness as a chronic pain and weakness in the lower back, with strain on one or more intervertebral disc. Eventually tissue deterioration ensues, and then problems with the discs and/or sacroiliac articulation become chronic.[33]

In the simplest sense, Rolfing will work first to bring length, space and resilience into the tissues. A strong, balanced base of support should be established in the feet. As mentioned in Chapter 5, *The Basic Ten-Session Series*, low back problems must be approached indirectly at first, slowly building session by session until there is the space and support to begin unwinding rotations.

I injured my back as a teenager by doing an incorrect front drop on a trampoline. I landed unevenly and hyperextended my lumbar vertebrae, wrenching the muscles of my lower back. Eventually the compression resulted in what was most likely a bulging disc between the 4th and 5th lumbar vertebrae that protruded anteriorly. In those days you didn't go to a doctor unless you were half-dead. As there were no broken bones, I was considered fine and continued on in my life with intermittent back pain. Being of good New England "grin and bear it" stock, I toughed out the pain during the bad times and forgot about it during the good times. When I encountered Rolfing in Tucson in 1976, I decided to get Rolfed more for the adventure of it than to relieve back pain. At the time, Rolfing was considered radical and "the thing to do" if you were on a growth path or working with humanistic psychology. Over the course of the Ten Sessions my weak and "accident prone" back began to get stronger and feel better. By the end of the Ten Series my back was probably fifty percent better and I had fewer relapses. But it was no miracle cure. Improvement occurred over many years of getting Rolfed and together with consciously working on changing my mental and physical habit patterns. Today I have only a slight shadow, now and then, of low back pain, just enough to keep me aware of when to stop certain activities. I can freely hike, bike, and do yoga with no pain, but believe me, it was a project. Typically, people hurt themselves, somewhat recover, and then forget about the original accident. When all of a sudden they begin to have chronic low back pain, they become mystified. Because of the way Rolfing works on overall patterns of stress in the myofascial system, problems of chronic low back pain are often relieved.

Whatever our particular process of making peace with the body looks like, we can be sure that we will be asked to accept ourselves as we are before we will be able to make any lasting changes in our outlook and in our behavior.
– CHRISTINA SELL, *YOGA FROM THE INSIDE OUT*, 96.

B.K.S. Iyengar mentions
that the brain is the
hardest part of the body
to adjust. Most people
believe that the brain is,
as he says, the subject –
in other words, the
source of consciousness.
But as he continues, our
brain and consciousness
are everywhere, diffuse
throughout our body,
and the "head" brain is
in fact an object of per-
ception, just like a leg or
an arm.
– RICHARD ROSEN THE
YOGA OF BREATH, 116.

Brain and Nervous System

We have already seen that, because of the physiological make up of the body, change on the surface radiates all the way to the cellular level. We have also considered that changes that affect the body also affect the mind, as mind and body are inseparable. Although Rolfers work primarily on the myofascial system of muscles and fascia and not directly with the nervous system, nonetheless Rolfers affect the nervous system indirectly, as James Oschman mentions here:

> We have described the fibrous systems in the connective tissue as a semiconductor communication network, and this applies to the collagenous fibers running through the vertebrae and the intervertebral discs. Hence alignment influences two kinds of communication: nerve impulses and semi conduction through the tensegrous network. Alignment of the collagenous networks has consequences for the overall energy field of the body.[34]

As the connective-tissue matrix supports and enfolds the nervous system, its nerves, and its plexi, affecting this matrix will affect what is within it. Most remarkable is that Rolfing, which is essentially addressing only the connective tissue that can be accessed through the hands, can actually change brain waves. According to Dr. Rolf, "...electroencephalographic (EEG) measurements have shown fundamental rhythm changes in brain waves long after initial manipulation work has been completed."[35] (More on this will be discussed in Chapter 12, *Research.*)

The nervous system is organized into three main branches:
- the central nervous system (CNS), consisting of the brain and spinal cord,
- the peripheral nervous system (PNS), which contains the cranial and spinal nerves,

- the autonomic nervous system (ANS), containing the sympathetic and parasympathetic branches.[36]

As mentioned previously, the autonomic nervous system is responsible for all of the basically unconscious bodily functions such as digestion, breathing, and heart rate. The sympathetic branch of the ANS gears up the body for action when danger is perceived – we have a response to flee or to fight. The parasympathetic branch of the ANS slows down bodily processes and generally calms the system. Many Rolfers have noticed the marked effect this work has on the autonomic nervous system. (More on this will be discussed in Chapter 11, *Trauma*.)

Robert Schleip, a Rolfer and Feldenkrais Practitioner, has done a masterful job of attempting to explain how Rolfing might work from a neural standpoint.

Fascia nevertheless is densely enervated by mechanoreceptors which are responsive to manual pressure. Stimulation of these sensory receptors has been shown to lead to a lowering of sympathetic tonus as well as a change in local viscosity. Additionally, smooth muscle cells have been discovered in fascia, which seem to be involved in active fascial contractility. Fascia and the autonomic nervous system appear to be intimately connected.[37]

Many of us (probably all of us) have had past traumas, both psychological and physical, that have over-activated the sympathetic branch of the ANS. This may be particularly true in situations where we were unable to flee or fight, and went instead into a freezing mode, such as in early childhood and birth trauma. The sympathetic branch of the ANS remains hyper-toned and thus we may be constantly tense, over alert, and ready for fight or flight. Schleip notes the benefits of steady, deep, manual pressure in calming sympathetic nervous system activity.

It therefore appears that deep manual pressure – specifically if it is slow or steady – stimulates interstitial and Ruffini mechanoreceptors, which results in an increase in vagal activity, which then changes not only local fluid dynamics and tissue metabolism, but also results in global muscle relaxation, as well as a more peaceful mind and less emotional arousal.[38]

I can feel this plasticity of the tissue when I am Rolfing. As I have mentioned previously, it feels like cold taffy that gets warmed up and then becomes stretchy and resilient. I also see and feel various responses from the autonomic nervous system in my clients. There are changes in breathing, sometimes a light sweat; the gut may begin to growl, or the body will have a fine almost invisible tremor. As I recorded in my class notes from Emmett Hutchins: if you don't see some autonomic response you're not getting deep enough into the system.

Of course the art of Rolfing is to put in enough information through the pressure of your hands to get deep change in the whole system, but not so much that the client is unable to receive and process that information. The Rolfer needs to develop a keen relationship with resistance – the resistance to change in the client and his or her tissue, and the Rolfer's own resistance to learning from the client. Force meeting resistance can involve an energetic standoff, like two rams butting heads. As a Rolfer I need to keep remembering that I am putting in information to a system that contains information to give back to me. It is quite a dance of walking along the edge!

Heart and Circulation
In considering what might happen in the heart and circulatory system when you get Rolfed, let's first consider that there are

two domains of "heart." There's the physiological heart that pumps blood through the blood vessels throughout the body, and then there's the heart as the seat of consciousness, spoken of so beautifully by the scientist Mae Wan Ho:

> Whenever people speak of "consciousness," they usually locate it to the brain, where ideas and intentions are supposed to flow, and which, through the nervous system, is supposed to control the entire body. I have always found that odd, for like all Chinese people, I was brought up on the idea that thoughts emanate from the heart.[39]

So many words are associated with the heart: such as, heartfelt, heart broken, a heart of gold. Here, of all places in the body, it is most difficult to pry the physiology apart from psychology. Heart rate can change with a mere thought. "We now know that each heartbeat begins with a pulse of electricity through the heart muscle…It is a basic law of physics that when an electrical current flows through a conductor, a magnetic field is created in surrounding space."[40] This electromagnetic field produced by the beating of the heart is measured by an electrocardiogram or ECG. And, while many electromagnetic fields are produced by the body, none is as strong as the field put out by the heart. This interplay of the two domains of heart becomes like the analogy of the shadow and the sun, causing us to ask where exactly does the shadow end and the sunlight begin? In this arena the boundary between the body and its environment begins to fade. "In the past we could define an individual as that which lies within the skin; but it is a fact of physics that energy fields are unbounded. The biomagnetic field of the heart extends indefinitely into space."[41]

One can only guess how the field of the heart interacts with the environment, whether it is other people, events, the gravitational field, or an unborn child. Joseph Chilton Pearce, in his

When you start to exert control over any bodily process, the effect is holistic. The mind-body system reacts to every single stimulus as a global event: i.e., to stimulate one cell is to stimulate all.

– DEEPAK CHOPRA M.D., *AGELESS BODY TIMELESS MIND*, 85.

book *The Biology of Transcendence*, describes an amazing experiment in which cells were taken from the heart of a live rodent (ouch!).

> We could take two live heart cells, keep them separated on the slide, and when fibrillation began, bring them closer together. At some magical point of spatial proximity they would stop fibrillating and resume their regular pulsing in synchrony with each other – a microscopic heart.[42]
>
> The same entrainment of heart frequencies occurs between mother and infant during breast feeding and other close body contact. Through this dynamic, the mother's developed heart furnishes the model frequencies that the infant's heart must have for its own development in the critical first months after birth.[43]

That kind of communication and intelligence in what many consider "just an organ" should give us pause. Needless to say, we want the heart to function well. In order to do this, the heart, like any other organ, needs space to function at its highest potential. Without the space, heart trouble can result, as Dr. Rolf confirmed to Peter Melchior when she first saw the structure of Fritz Perls (the founder of Gestalt therapy). Peter remembers how Dr. Rolf said, "Well no wonder the man's having heart attacks. Look at the left side of his chest. It's all caved in."[44] As Peter reported in Chapter 1 on Dr. Rolf, after Perls received about twelve Rolfing sessions from Dr. Rolf, he was able to walk up the hill at Esalen without becoming so out of breath he had to keep stopping. Perls was impressed enough with the improvement he felt that he started sending his students to get Rolfed by Dr. Rolf.

In considering circulation, visualize a huge network of veins, arteries and capillaries spreading throughout the body, embedded in fascia, snaking through and in between muscles and organs, carrying nutrients to every cell, organ and muscle. This ultimate "postal service" of the body, the circulatory system, carries information ceaselessly to every tissue and cell of the body while we sit and read a book, oblivious to this ongoing wonder. Imagine if these channels and tubes of bloodflow become pressed on and blocked by twisted, misplaced and hardened connective tissue. The flow will become more sluggish, and so will all bodily functions. With Rolfing, as the muscles become more elastic and move in their proper relationships, the exchange of metabolites and waste products at the cellular level increases. As Dr. Rolf explained:

> In any living body, a change in the metabolic efficiency, to be significant, must occur at the cellular level (in the ground substance of the interstitial tissue), not merely in the chemical contents of the blood as it circulates. Muscles are important pumping mechanisms for this process. When their balance in space is appropriate, their capacity for their particular work is good; they will be resilient and elastic and their function of flooding and draining tissue will be effective.[45]

Our own physical body possesses a wisdom which we who inhabit the body lack. We give it orders which make no sense.
— HENRY MILLER

To put it most simply, I am always aiming to "get something moving" when I Rolf someone. Life is movement, and every part of the body should be able to freely move. When I place my hands on the body and press into the connective tissue web, I am first asking for a response of subtle movement. When muscles and fascia begin to stretch, all heaven and hell break loose. Some organization is needed. We must first create space so there can be movement, then we need to organize the tissue around a central principle (the Rolf Line) so that all these ongoing, diverse, yet intricately related, systems can function as they were designed.

*If all people learned
to think in the
non-Aristotelian manner
of quantum mechanics,
the world would change
so radically that most of
what we call "stupidity"
and even a great deal of
what we consider "insan-
ity" might disappear,
and the "intractable"
problems of war,
poverty and injustice
would suddenly seem
a great deal closer to
solution.*

— ALFRED KORZYBSKI

Both Mae Wan Ho and Candace Pert mentioned a harmonious set of interrelationships in the body that function like a symphony. Varied instruments harmonize into one whole that is far greater than the sum of its parts. Getting Rolfed, you have the potential to become a living symphony – a being that radiates harmony, beauty and well being. Those of us who get Rolfed become an ongoing part of Dr. Rolf's experiment in what happens when humans become aligned around a principle of verticality.

The Psychological Aspect of the Body-Mind

In her classes Dr. Rolf often mentioned the work of Alfred Korzybski – who formulated a new way of speaking and thinking, which he called "general semantics." Korzybski's book, *Science and Sanity*, was first published in 1933. The breadth and scholarly detail of this massive small-print tome is staggering. Looking through this book one can see why Dr. Rolf might have been interested in such an innovative thinker. In the preface to his second edition Korzybski wrote:

General semantics is not any "philosophy," or "psychology," or "logic," in the ordinary sense. It is a new extensional discipline which explains and trains us how to use our nervous systems most efficiently…In brief, it is the formulation of a new non-Aristotelian system of orientation which affects every branch of science and life.[46]

Korzybski then went on to speak of:

…a new functional definition of 'man', formulated in 1921, based on an analysis of uniquely human *potentialities*; namely that each generation may begin where the former left off. This characteristic I called the "time binding" capacity. Here the reactions of humans are not split verbally and elementalistically into separate "body," "mind," "emotions," "intellect," "intuitions," etc., but are treated from an organism-as-a-whole-in-an-environment (*external and internal*) point of view.[47]

With a bold yet detailed brushstroke, Korzybski was setting out to develop a new theory of how to think about the human being – seeing him less from cause and effect, than in sets of relationships; less in pieces and more as a whole.

In the first chapter of her book *Rolfing: The Integration of Human Structures*, Dr. Rolf delves into this idea of seeing the human as a whole and sets up her premise regarding the relationship between behavior and physiology.

One of the pregnant ideas of this decade [1970s] is that human behavior is basically an outward and visible functional response of structural organization (or lack of it). This idea (traditionally called *monism*) is not making its bow for the first time. One modern reincarnation of monism is psychosomatic medicine. Within this particular framework, psychotherapy again postulates that our external circumstances are projections of our internal being.[48]

"The body is the unconscious mind!,"[49] Dr. Candace Pert has said; and twenty years earlier Dr. Rolf was saying, "Emotional response is behavior, is function. All behavior is expressed through the musculoskeletal system. All function is an expression of structure and form and correlates directly with material structure. A man crying the blues is in reality bewailing his structural limitations and failures."[50]

My class notes from Emmett Hutchins report that Dr. Rolf has referred to the connective tissue system as the organ that connects soma to psyche; the material to the non-material; and that one can affect a person's emotional and causal bodies through connective tissue.[51] Rolfing is one of the more powerful methods for affecting deeply-held patterns of behavior directly through physical reorganization of the myofascial system.

The "Chicken and Egg" of Psychology and Physiology

When there is physical trauma to the body, emotional behavior will express that trauma. Likewise, when there is emotional trauma, this is also expressed in the body. Whether the physical or the mental-emotional aspect of a person first becomes unbalanced, these patterns become locked in the flesh, and each perpetuates the other until there is an inseparable relationship between bodily expression and mental-emotional expression of these patterns. When, for example, five-year-old Bobby reacts to the emotional trauma of psychological abuse by a parent, he may become angry and aggressive. He may pull up his shoulders, restrict his breathing, round his arms forward to protect his heart, and stiffen his body in preparation to defend himself. This pattern of response then becomes locked in his body; thirty years later he may wonder why he is having a hard time with personal relationships. Bobby's flesh is now fixed and hard, interfering with the flow of fluids and energy throughout his body. He feels constantly threatened and on edge and doesn't know why. He may end up going to a psychotherapist, but the going will be slow and difficult. As long as his physical structure is hard, unyielding and in a defensive pattern, it will be next to impossible for his inner experience – and his outwardly expressed behavior to change in any deep and permanent way. His psychological patterns are literally embodied in the flesh.

I find this totally fascinating. The fact that I am placing my hands directly on a psychological pattern that is manifested physically, and can be worked with so directly through the re-organization of connective tissue, is nothing short of amazing. Don't get me wrong, however. Even though I have a degree in counseling and a background in Gestalt therapy, I don't stop in the middle of a Rolfing session and do psychotherapy. If needed, I will refer my client to a psychotherapist. Psychotherapy and Rolfing work very well together as the Rolfing begins to open up old, stuck patterns of emotional behavior. It is enough to keep my client focused on the "now" of his or her body sensation, and to keep her physical structure as balanced as possible during a Rolfing session.

I have clearly experienced how much physical imbalance affects one's emotional state. Once, in class, after being worked on by my class partner, I felt totally weepy and fragile. Tom Wing came over and gave me a specific, integrating move that settles the sacrum and integrates changes through the spine. Immediately I felt fine. At other times in class I noticed how powerful the integrating moves were at helping the client to feel emotionally strong, grounded, and ready to move out into the world. When emotions come up in the middle of the Rolfing session and I have only completed one side of the body, my first job is to be present with the client and Rolf the other side of the body!

Working with Embedded Patterns

When "Allan" – a client with whom I worked off and on for about seven years – first came to me he was complaining of pain in his hips and legs that was curtailing his physical workouts. He'd just been divorced, was working in a job he didn't like, and was living in a small, dingy apartment. Allan constantly complained about his life and seemed genuinely at a loss as to why his wife might have left him. The fact that he might have had any responsibility for the divorce completely eluded him.

Allan's body was extremely rigid, with overdeveloped muscles and little flexibility. Even his workout schedule was rigid – exact

According to energy medicine, we are all living history books. Our bodies contain our histories – every chapter, line and verse of every event and relationship in our lives. As our lives unfold, our biological health becomes a living, breathing biographical statement that conveys our strengths, weaknesses, hopes and fears.

– CAROLINE MYSS, PH.D., ANATOMY OF THE SPIRIT, 40.

timings, an exact number of repetitions, and a sense of failure if he didn't meet the goals he had set. Allan's pattern was to feel as though his environment and everyone in it was conspiring against him. He had trouble feeling his body unless it was in pain. Allan was one unhappy guy.

Over the years that I was Rolfing him, Allan made dramatic changes. As his body softened and lengthened, and as he had less and less pain, his whole attitude began to slowly shift. He became lighter, and his inherent sense of humor began to emerge. Allan became more permeable, flexible and resilient, not only in his body, but in his personality, which made him much more fun to be around. During the seven years that I knew him, Allan became a partner in his own lucrative company, bought a beautiful house, and remarried. I certainly could not say that *because* Allan was Rolfed *therefore* he made these profound life changes. Yet, when you consider that the physical structure and the expression of that structure are not two separate things, I can assert that there is tremendous possibility for change in emotional expression from a reordering of the body.

Dr. Rolf used to say that we were educators rather than therapists, and I find that the Rolfing process is a wonderful arena for unobtrusively teaching my clients through their newly-found awareness in their bodies. They seem to be able to assimilate more easily the metaphors in their bodies that speak of psychological patterns they may not ordinarily wish to see. For the client to discover by direct physical experience that she is holding her breath, and that right now it is O.K. to breathe fully, can be much less threatening for her than verbally digging into her past and discovering the trauma that might be hidden there.

My client "Samantha" provides a good example of my being able to use the Rolfing process to teach new patterns of behavior directly, through her own developing awareness of her body. Samantha was a downhill ski racer in her teenage years. During that time she had two severe sprains, one of her left ankle, and one of her left knee. She also had a fall that injured her low back, leaving her with intermittent low back spasms. As none of those injuries were fractures, Samantha continued on with her skiing and athletics, setting up a pattern of favoring her left ankle and knee, eventually resulting in a rotation of her pelvis and a serious compromise to her skiing technique. Over time she developed a feeling of insecurity and fear of failure, as her body refused to perform at the level she wished in her competitive sports. Samantha began to feel like life was a struggle to "win" and that she was not good enough – not good enough to win in sports, and not good enough to win love. She expressed this pattern of insecurity with a collapsed chest, a heavy ungrounded walk, a lack of physical awareness, and a fogginess of presence as if she wasn't quite all here.

During her Rolfing sessions I worked a lot on Samantha's legs, feet and hips, beginning to teach her how to tune in to her body, as she became more supported and grounded in her physical structure. Samantha had a habit pattern of assuming the worst, and would begin to withdraw almost before I touched her. I called her attention to her bodily sensation as we worked, and taught her how to drop her attention deeper and connect her awareness from where I was directly working to another related place in her body.

Samantha was especially challenging and fun to work with, as she was enthusiastic about the Rolfing and ready for change. As her physical structure became stronger and more balanced, she grew in confidence, and her habitual patterns of withdrawal were revealed to her during the Rolfing sessions. I could then use the pressure of my hand, or the small movements I might ask her to make, as teaching tools to give her an opportunity to successfully move through some of her fear. By sensing exactly how she was holding and withdrawing, Samantha could then make a choice to *use* the sensation of my touch to become more present.

Illness becomes a process and not an event. If a person can be shown how an accident or illness can serve as a teacher, the accident or illness can actually assume a role in the evolution and growth of the individual.
– FRITZ FREDERICK SMITH, M.D., *INNER BRIDGES*, 17.

Although I have personally received a great deal of excellent psychotherapy and certainly made some mental changes in myself, when I look back on my life, getting Rolfed was the beginning of a new level of change, and a powerful influence on my expression of who I am. It's hard to express joy, spontaneity, serenity or confidence in an unbalanced vehicle locked up with past personal history. It's hard to let go of that personal history if it is physically retained in the body. The cells literally carry memory of trauma, and there have been many times when my clients have suddenly remembered a childhood trauma during a Rolfing session. You have to know the wound is there before it can be healed.

Cellular memory is truly amazing. Once, during a Rolfing session on my feet and legs, I remembered the exact time, place and feeling of the day I was flying down a ski hill with some friends when a slower skier turned right in front of me. I was forced to crash into the woods, badly spraining my ankle. During the Rolfing, I could feel how I had favored this ankle, and now I was able to move it in a different way. Afterwards, I could bear full weight on it again. Before that particular Rolfing session, I had forgotten all about that ankle sprain, as it had become so deeply embedded in my system.

The Teachers Speak about What Happens When You Get Rolfed

Having looked at some possible physiological and psychological, or body-mind, aspects of what might be happening when you get Rolfed, let's hear from my four teachers about how Rolfing might work.

Emmett Hutchins

Primarily I think it [Rolfing] works because that's the way the structure would like to be anyway…[Dr. Rolf] implied

My body is the fundamental matrix within which I experience the world. On the basis of my experience, I participate with others in creating the larger structures of the world: social, economic, political, artistic. When the structure of my body changes, my experience changes, thus changing my relationship to other structures.

– DON JOHNSON, THE PROTEAN BODY, 116.

to me many years ago that…there would be a time when a person would get enough order that it would create more order…on its own. About four years ago I began to experience that, and I think that many people could experience it much earlier than I did. I had a body filled with a lot of scar tissue, [and] two major traumas…[Even though] I've gotten less work on my own body in the last two years than I did the previous five, I've had more changes…I'm at the place where I…feel like just putting in my Line [the Rolf Line] every day brings on a new layer of awareness, and then something new happens every single day whether anybody works with me or not. There are enough things right in my structure now that they're able to win over any kind of an argument with something that's wrong, assuming that I don't step off the curb wrong and really mess myself up badly.

That's the wonderful gift of paying attention to my Line for all these years…A body has its own auto-immune system and its own way of fighting disease and its own way of nutrition and its own way of communing with the divine mind; it is the most fantastic playground and laboratory and invention in the whole world and we are all part of it. And so…what makes this [Rolfing] work is that I think Structural Integration just simply gives you a body to communicate with reality. This is a structure [that] is not fighting its existence so much. It is being supported by the universe and as a result it functions better; it fights disease better; it digests food better; it works better; it doesn't have as many negative moods; it isn't offended by other events as much. There's just no thing that doesn't get improved with a structure that doesn't experience some kind of constant irritation.[52]

* * *

Over the years there has been much discussion among Rolfers about the physiological aspect of change that we referred to as "gel to sol" – a concept that Dr. Rolf often mentioned in her classes. This concept was based on the chemical changes that happen in connective tissues when energy is added. The collagen fibers that make up fascia are imbedded in a ground substance that is a semi-fluid called "gel."[53] As to how such rapid changes to connective tissues might be occurring with Rolfing, Dr. Rolf theorized:

> The continuous metabolic interchange made possible through the intimate relation of fascia with water metabolism allows structural reorganization…the speed so clearly apparent in fascial change must be a property of its complex ground substance. The universal distribution of connective tissue calls attention to the likelihood that this colloidal gel is the universal internal environment. Every living cell seems to be in contact with it, and its modification under changes of pressure would account for the wide spectrum of effects seen in Structural Integration. The application of pressure is, in fact, the addition of energy to the tissue colloid. (It is well known in physics that the addition of energy can turn colloid gel into sol.)[54]

The sensation for both Rolfer and client is a softening of the tissues and thus the word "sol" (or solution), as it is described chemically above. In the interview material that follows, the shortcut description of this possible theory is referred to as "gel sol."

Peter Melchoir

I don't think we [really know what's happening on a physiological level]. I don't think we're even close. There are a lot of people who have a lot of different ideas about it, and oddly enough they all work. Who knows?

Regarding the theory of "gel-sol," Peter believed it was an honest attempt to try to find a possible explanation for what was happening – for what we could see and feel – in the fascia.

That ["gel-sol"] was the idea she came up with for something that was happening in the [cellular] matrix. It's still not a bad idea. It's just that something tells me it's not exactly that simple. I think we have to look at the psychophysical. I think it's the leading edge of where we are as a culture. We don't know [exactly how Rolfing works]. It's been shown dramatically in some cases, certainly in healing, that there are all kinds of things that happen that have nothing to do with the plain, straight physical.[55]

Jan Sultan

One contextual thing is that Rolf told us that before she got to Esalen she really saw her work as an adjunct to orthopedics. It was only after her interception with Esalen that she began to get into the human potential side. So, having said that, I think some of what makes it [Rolfing] really work is the systematic decompensation of historic adaptive patterning. Nobody else tried to do a global repatterning the way Rolf did...[There is also the] external referent of gravity as the template for the repatterning. You weren't just unstressing the body but you were going toward a new pattern, which Rolf said was defined by gravity's influence on the body. Huge! [The] external referent of gravity [is] the template for the repatterning. [There is also] the plasticity of fascia which is that ["gel to sol"] thing that she [Dr. Rolf] talked about so much."

Specifically regarding the "gel-sol" theory, Jan says:

Energy is the real substance behind the appearance of matter and forms.

– RANDOLPH STONE, D.O., D.C., N.D.

"Well, I sort of have one foot still in it. The other foot is really in a whole other domain, which is the orienting and righting reflexes that get repatterned when you change shape. Then there's the Golgi tendon-organ-muscle spindle reflex interaction – so that when you change the tonus in the ligament bed, muscles change tone. I actually think in some way she [Dr. Rolf] didn't really get that piece because she didn't emphasize it in her training and it was only later when Robert Schleip started to really campaign this that I got it. But the Golgi tendon-organ reflex arc…is linked with fundamental righting reflex and orientation patterning. So, when you get into the fascia and the ligament bed you're in the brain stem and the hypothalamus. That's why that…really change[s] how we handle ourselves.

Our fundamental sense of self is linked to spatial organization – how we experience ourselves. So that if you can change someone's spatial orientation and the way that they maintain their space literally, you also have openings in the development of the character that can be exploited – the "who am I" question. The touch [of Rolfing] is fundamentally a kind of education that happens below the mind so it's not cognitive, it's actually sensation driven. That's also really important.[56]

Tom Wing

That's all true [gel to sol theory] *and*…in my mind, that's a good story to tell to explain the phenomena. I think there are other stories as well. I think there are different stories that can explain it. I don't trust one story line anymore. One time Ida got upset with somebody because they kept saying, "Why? Why this? Why that?" And Ida said, "*Why* is not a useful question. The only answer to why is *because*. If you are going to have one *because*, you are going to have

to have at least a dozen, because one will never cover it."
And I think it's the same here; it's like what makes it
[Rolfing] work is a *why*. Why does it work? Because it
does."

Another piece of it for me is that I think it [Rolfing]
works to the degree in which it is congruent with the
processes of the body in its desire to improve its integration – to become more integrated and more balanced and
freer. I think it works in direct proportion to how relevant
what's being done at the moment is to the process within
the organism itself. The degree to which you vary from
that diminishes the results. That doesn't say how it works,
but that's my belief on it.

I also think that [how Rolfing works] is still a mystery.
I think that's still a question to ask ourselves all the time
because I don't think we still know the answer, just [as] we
don't know the answer to the question, "What is Rolfing?"
There's another good one for you! Ida refused to answer
that one. At this point in life I am more [interested in just
doing the Rolfing] than I am in trying to figure it out. It's
sort of like...living the question. I don't know how it
works; I don't know why it works.[57]

*But the body is deeper
than the soul and its
secrets inscrutable.*
– E. M. FORSTER

* * *

What happened for me when I got Rolfed? I woke up; I learned
how to feel my body again, to be present, and to get my feet on the
ground and my eyes open. My body became my friend instead of a
painful hunk of flesh from which I was trying to escape. Though it
took years, my back pain is gone, and my scoliosis is moveable,
pain free, and integrated into my system. Rolfing became not only
my profession, but a way of life.

SARAH'S STORY

I interviewed Sarah many years after her first Ten Sessions of Rolfing. Beyond this, she received additional Rolfing both from me and from Peter Melchior. Her story is particularly interesting because it takes a long view of her life – we learn about the paths she chose to take after her initial Rolfing. Sarah is quite articulate, and expresses some of the broader reaches of Rolfing. At the time of her initial Ten-Session Series, Sarah was a young mother with four children. She had married shortly after graduation from college and was fairly consumed with her marriage and children. She first heard about Rolfing because her sister was studying to be a Rolfer at the time.

As soon as I experienced the first session, and even when I first heard what it was about, I thought Rolfing might be a fascinating journey. I had no idea what a big one it would be. As soon as I started, I realized that I was not in touch with my body, particularly due to being married and having four children over a fairly short period of time. I felt like I had been a vehicle for all those births – I had been nursing children and I didn't really know who I was and sort of how I fit in space.

When I started Rolfing, my youngest child was just entering kindergarten, and this meant a shift of my role, as I wasn't needed on a daily basis. A big shift! I was ready to explore what my next step was. I felt like Rolfing was considerably bigger than I had originally thought; I never dreamed that the body could change so much. It was pretty mind boggling.

WHAT HAPPENS WHEN YOU GET ROLFED? 171

I had a lot of discomfort when the actual work was being done in certain places, and then I felt the freedom when that particular move ended and I could "fill up" the new space that was created.

Sarah had to drive two hours to get to her Rolfer, and then after each session she had to drive home and reenter her life as mother and wife. Originally she and her husband had planned to receive the Rolfing together, but he changed his mind. For Sarah, the changes she was experiencing in herself needed to be integrated back into her family life. The integration of changes that take place in the body is as large a piece of the work as the initial physical and emotional shifts are. Sarah had a particularly challenging time with this, as parts of herself that she had kept hidden were now emerging.

There were times that it was particularly difficult to come back into my home environment after having had such a huge piece of work, and to not talk about it too much because it was a little hard to translate. I had to play the dance of not admitting that I was changing quite as much as I was. I had my…spiritual self always kind of tucked away, maybe ready to go to when I wanted to, but I didn't have to manifest it in my daily life.

It was O.K. for me to live that way. The process of Rolfing brought those parts of myself more together, and it brought this sort of spiritual-seeker part more present in my flesh, so that it was harder to compartmentalize my life.

The thread common to all spiritual myths is that human beings are compelled to merge our bodies with the essence of God, that we want to have the Divine in our bones and blood and in our mental and emotional makeup. In belief systems around the world, conceptions of the Divine's spiritual nature reflect the best human qualities and characteristics.

– CAROLINE MYSS, PH.D., ANATOMY OF THE SPIRIT, 66.

Also, I do remember feeling, at that time, that this was a road from which I couldn't turn back. I think that's the other thing about memorable sessions – feeling off balance in between, and looking forward to the next piece of work. Because one thing would shift and the other part would not feel quite right. But even the times when I would feel unbalanced, I was so excited about the change that it felt like an adventure that I was choosing to go on.

The adventure Sarah was choosing to go on turned out to be a divorce from her husband and a subsequent change in the direction of her life from wife and mother, to mother and professional educator and healer. Over the ensuing years, Sarah received a master's degree in education and became a certified massage therapist, Zero Balancing® practitioner, and craniosacral therapist. She presently teaches reading recovery at the elementary level, and practices massage, Zero Balancing, and craniosacral work.

In looking back over the years since she first was Rolfed, Sarah described the effect of Rolfing in her life as follows:

I think it was the biggest life-changing experience I've had so far in terms of...blowing my cover. Really, it was about me coming into more of who I really am – definitely empowering, definitely freeing. In the beginning [it was] sort of a long journey of potential, of opening doors to the fact that this was an ongoing process and that one of the best ways for me to work on my emotional self was through the body. I think that this is definitely the stuff of the spirit…There is incredible potential for human growth in the process of Rolfing.

I see similar things happening over and over again in the lives of my clients. You couldn't prove it scientifically, but when a person becomes more who she or he really is, she is less apt to put up with relationships, jobs, and patterns of life that are not in line with who she is becoming. My final question to Sarah was: "So it sounds like you're saying that your most memorable experience about Rolfing was much more about growth and evolution, that kind of thing, than fixing a sore back." She replied, "Absolutely." I have actually fixed her sore back a couple of times when it has gone out. Of course she wanted to be out of pain and able to function again, but most of all I think she wanted to be able to continue on her journey.

Endnotes, Chapter 6

[1] Rolf, Ida P. "Rolfing Structural Integration: Gravity: An Unexplored Factor in the More Human Use of Human Beings." *The Journal of the Institute for the Comparative Study of History, Philosophy and the Sciences.* Vol. I, Number 1, June Issue, 1963, 7. This article was copyrighted by Dr. Rolf in 1962 and reprinted by the Rolf Institute.
[2] Feitis, Rosemary. Editor. *Ida Rolf Talks About Rolfing and Physical Reality.* New York, N.Y.: Harper and Row, 1978, 41.
[3] Pearce, Joseph Chilton. *The Biology of Transcendence: A Blueprint of the Human Spirit.* Rochester, Vermont: Park Street Press, 2002, 87.
[4] Ho, Mae Wan. *The Rainbow and the Worm: The Physics of Organisms Second Edition.* New Jersey: World Scientific Publishing Company, 1998, 174.
[5] Rolf, 7.
[6] Ibid., 6.

[7] Pert, Candace B. *The Molecules of Emotion: Why You Feel the Way You Feel.* New York, N.Y.: Scribner, 1997, 130.

[8] Ibid., 141.

[9] Ho, Mae Wan, 185, 186.

[10] Ibid., 185. Ho credits Oschman as follows in her footnote – Oschman, J.W. "Structure and Properties of Ground Substances." *American Zoologist* 24:199-215, 1984.

[11] Feitis, 124.

[12] Ida P. Rolf. Rolf class notes.

[13] Oschman, James H., Ph.D."What is Healing Energy? The Scientific Basis of Energy Medicine." From a series of articles published in the *Journal of Bodywork and Movement Therapies*. Edited by Leon Chaitow, N.D, D.O, New York, N.Y.: Churchill Livingstone, 1996-1998, 300.

[14] Kirkby, Ron Ph.D."The Probably Reality Behind Structural Integration: How Gravity Supports the Body." Paper written for a Rolfing class and reprinted by The Rolf Institute of Structural Integration, undated, 2.

[15] Ibid., 4.

[16] Ibid., 4.

[17] Ibid., 10.

[18] Ibid., 10.

[19] Ho, Mae Wan, 85.

[20] Ibid., 185. Ho credits Donald Ingber as follows: Ingber, D.E. "The Riddle of Morphogenesis: A Question of Solution Chemistry or Molecular Cell Engineering?" *Cell* 75 (1993): 1249-52.

[21] Hutchins, Emmett. Interview. Kauai, Hawaii. June 9, 2004.

[22] Pert, 186, 187.

[23] Feitis, 129.

[24] Fulford, Robert C. D.O. with Gene Stone. *Dr. Fulford's Touch of Life: The Healing Power of the Natural Life Force.* New York, N.Y.: Pocket Books, A division of Simon and Schuster, Inc. 1996, 41.

[25] Feitis, 168, 169.

[26] Rolf, Ida P. Ph.D. *Rolfing: The Integration of Human Structures.* Santa Monica, California: Dennis-Landman, 1977, 65.

[27] Ibid., 113.

[28] Ibid., 113.

[29] Pert, 188.

[30] Ibid., 188.

[31] Rolf, *Rolfing: The Integration of Human Structures*, 187.

[32] Ibid., 143.

[33] Ibid., 79.

34 Oschman, 1.

35 Rolf, *Rolfing: The Integration of Human Structures*, 202.

36 Watson, Craig MD, and Ph.D. *Basic Human Neuroanatomy: An Introductory Atlas Second Edition*. Boston, Massachusetts: Little, Brown and Company, 1977, 3.

37 Schleip, Robert, M.A. "Fascial Plasticity- A New Neurobiological Explanation Part I." *The 2004 Yearbook of Structural Integration*. Missoula, Montana: The International Association of Structural Integrators, 2004, 64.

38 Ibid., 69.

39 Ho, Mae Wan. 185.

40 Oschman, 118.

41 Ibid.

42 Pearce, Joseph Chilton. *The Biology of Transcendence: A Blueprint of the Human Spirit*. Rochester, Vermont: Park Street Press, 2002, 55.

43 Ibid., 60 – 61.

44 Melchior, Peter. Interview. Lyons, Colorado. March 4, 2004.

45 Rolf, *Rolfing: The Integration of Human Structures*, 51.

46 Korzybski, Alfred. *Science and Sanity: An Introduction to Non-Aristotelian Systems and General Semantics 4ᵗʰ Edition*. Lakeville, Connecticut: The International Non-Aristotelian Library Publishing Company, 1958, xxvi, xxvii.

47 Ibid., xx.

48 Rolf, Ida P. Ph.D. *Rolfing: The Integration of Human Structures*, 21.

49 Pert, Candace B. *The Molecules of Emotion: Why You Feel the Way You Feel*. New York, N.Y.: Scribner, 1997, 141.

50 Rolf, Ida P. Ph.D. *Rolfing: The Integration of Human Structures*, 17.

51 Hutchins, Emmett. Rolf class notes.

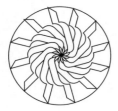

7
The Issue of Pain

Often when people first hear the word "Rolfing" they also hear that it is painful. Let's look at what pain *is*, exactly.

A physiology textbook – such as Watson's *Basic Human Neuroanatomy: An Introductory Atlas* – offers a long, involved definition, referring to a somatic-afferent nerve pathways from receptors moving through synapses and on into the spinal cord ending in the parietal lobe of the cerebral cortex.[1] Pain's scope is touched upon in Ganong's *Review of Medical Physiology 7th Edition*, which states: "The sense organs for pain are the naked nerve endings found in almost every tissue of the body."[2] In the most basic and practical sense, pain is information – a sensation that demands attention.

Certainly pain has a complicated physiologic pathway, but because the brain and emotions are involved, we humans can directly affect how we perceive pain. As much as thirty years ago, this psychic-emotional component was noted in Ganong's basic physiology book, in which he wrote: "Pain was called by Sherrington the 'psychical adjunct of an imperative protective reflex.' Stimuli which are painful generally initiate potent withdrawal and avoidance responses. Furthermore pain is peculiar among the sens-es in that it is associated with a strong emotional component."[3]

With the groundbreaking work of neuroscientist Candace Pert, Ph.D., and her discovery of what she called "the molecules of emotion," the meaning of pain takes on a whole new dimen-sion. In her book *The Molecules of Emotion: Why You Feel the Way You Feel*, Pert corroborates some of the things Dr. Rolf was tossing about in her own mind about the interrelationship of mind and body, when she writes, "The body is the unconscious mind! Repressed traumas caused by overwhelming emotion can be stored in a body part, thereafter affecting our ability to feel that part or even move it."[4] When that buried trauma, which is literally stored in the muscles, is contacted by a Rolfer's touch, the client may feel an intense sensation that might be referred to as "pain." (This will be discussed more in Chapter 11, *Trauma*.)

Pain *is* peculiar, because to some degree we have a choice as to how to respond to it. Once, at Esalen Institute, I attended a class involving hypnosis. When the participants were deeply relaxed, we were asked if we wanted to try an experiment. I raised my hand and was given a clamp, of the type that is used to close off arteries during surgery, and told to put this clamp on the back of my hand. I remember so clearly being surprised that this registered only as strong sensation. As everything was slowed down, I had a choice of how I could receive and interpret this input. Through past experience I was tempted to tighten up and feel this as pain, but in that moment I chose to stay relaxed and simply watch the sen-sation. Later, when we were all in a normal state, the clamps were passed around again. This time when I fastened it onto the back of my hand I felt instant and strong pain and had to immediately remove the clamp.

Your body is your history of your unique path of avoiding pain.
– DON JOHNSON, THE PROTEAN BODY, 48.

Pain and Rolfing

Change itself can be painful. At a deep level, most of us don't want to change. When a force for change meets up with resistance, the intent to withdraw is usually present and, as Ida Rolf stated, that drawing back results in pain.

Rolfing is about change. It's intent is to change structure, and such change is not always a walk in the park! As any change can be painful – whether it is a move, a new job, a need to alter attitudes or psychological patterns, or the end (or beginning) of a relationship – "painless Rolfing" would be an oxymoron. While it would be great if Rolfing or any other change were painless, it can't be guaranteed. Emmett Hutchins had this to say about pain in general, and specifically in the early days of Rolfing:

The motor intent to remove the body from a sensation is pain.
    – IDA P. ROLF

I don't think it [pain] was ever one of her [Dr. Rolf's] main concerns, nor has it ever been one of mine. Pain was one of those unavoidable things. I think she allowed us to create a lot more pain than necessary, and knowingly. She knew of no other way to get us into the body to the point where [we would] get enough familiarity to know how to treat people. We were all totally ignorant when it came to changing deep structure and deep places in structure. So, she would let us cause a great deal of discomfort (and unnecessary discomfort I think) because she felt that that would be our avenue for learning to do what we had to do. But pain was never a consideration.

I've always felt that pain was a nuisance and that if I really knew how to do it right, it [Rolfing] wouldn't be painful. I'm always looking for a less painful way to do things, a more comfortable way to do things, and so I always consider pain to be a negative. But, I'd much rather cause pain and get the job done. So I have never avoided doing something just because of the pain if I thought it was going to be useful.[5]

Tom Wing came to similar conclusions as he worked in his own practice:

Well, the way I came to it [this issue of pain] from my own understanding that whenever there's pain there's resistance,...they go together. I'm not going to say one is causal but they go together...my hands told me that whenever anyone reported pain there was resistance in the tissue. That always was so. So I began to explore that correlation. Could I train myself to say, "When I feel *this* I know that there's resistance; and [when] I feel this level of resistance I suspect that [the client is] feeling what somebody would call 'pain'?"

Different people have different interpretations [of pain] and, in my own process, part of the whole pain thing was learning discrimination and differentiation. When I started my Rolfing I had two categories: it feels good or it hurts; if it doesn't feel good it must be pain.

[The issue of pain] is an ongoing exploration in trying to come to my own sense of differentiation of stimuli, my interpretation of those stimuli, and [my experience in] how I work[ed] with that on the personal level. My response to an *intense* experience might be different than my response to a *painful* experience. In my mind I would go, "Oh this is pain. This is to be avoided. It's to be gotten away from. It's got to be stopped." Whereas something intense is, "Well, that's to be worked with."[6]

Suffering is drawing back.

— IDA P. ROLF

Working with pain is a dance, a contact improvisation between Rolfer and client. When my clients ask about the issue of pain, I tell them that we can work in such a way that it doesn't have to be a problem. If a client is tense and actively withdrawing, she is not working with or accepting and being present with what is going on. I try not to put in more information than the client can assimilate in that moment. This involves a sensitive and aware touch, and a keen interaction with the client. I want to challenge the client to change without her having to tense up and withdraw.

I teach my clients how to be present with the sensation, and try to give them a sensation with which they can work. It is *very* tempting to back off from this challenge and just make the client comfortable. Sometimes I do back off – it depends on the client's pathology and their ability to work. The bottom line for me is to work in such a way as to teach the client to be aware of *sensation* and to learn to see that they don't have to be afraid of it – that there are many kinds of sensations, and that it is all interesting information for them to have.

The key that I have learned over the years is to not try to push through resistance, but to go right up against it so that the client can feel it, yet still be able to stay present without withdrawing. Then, if I wait right there at that edge of resistance where the client can be present with me, the tissue begins to soften and stretch. As I take my hands off, the client often feels a new sense of ease and space in that area, and is thus encouraged to move on.

"Judy" described her learning process regarding pain:

I had a lot of past conditioning that good things didn't come without pain and that you needed to be tough and so I was going to be the toughest and I was certainly not going to complain…I think that my Rolfer *did* work with me on how to go into the pain and use it. But, there were times [when] I was a little over the edge on being able to handle it. But then when the Rolfing stopped, and I felt so

Energetically, pain is caused by movement being blocked.
– Fritz Frederick Smith, M.D., *Inner Bridges*, 142.

good, then I wanted to come back for more. So it felt that [the pain] was a necessary part of the process.

My experience with the pain of Rolfing has definitely shifted as I've received advanced Rolfing. I'm [also] able to work within my own body more efficiently. Particularly my experience with…[my Rolfer] telling me to go to another place [and] to let go of it where the other end of the string is [see below for explanation]. It was hugely valuable to me and the Rolfing has never been as painful since I learned to sink into the connections of the body more.

What Judy meant by the "string" imagery was that the Rolfer is able to feel tension in another part of the connective tissue system – a part that is related to the area being worked on. By suggesting that Judy place her attention on that other area – "where the other end of the string is" – she releases her resistance in the area being worked on and thus feels less pain. Judy went on to articulate her experience of being Rolfed by an advanced practitioner, Peter Melchior:

It was deep structural change without pain, and it felt like he was accessing all levels at the same time, and that's why it all moved a little easier.

The other feeling I had with Peter's touch was that it was deep but very caring and gentle. That's not to say that the other Rolfing I received wasn't caring and gentle. The biggest piece was the way it felt like he could see all of me at once, or feel all of me at once, and that was really huge. I definitely experienced the session as a kind of a sacred experience that one could be that deeply connected with somebody and they could work with you on that level and that it could actually be easy, which was so against my childhood programming…After that experience with

Peter…I began to shift to be able to experience Rolfing in a different way. I wasn't expecting [any longer] that one of the main things I had to do was suffer.

Learning from Pain

Dr. Rolf suggested that the wider the range of stimuli you can recognize and assimilate into the organism, the less fear there will be around a particular sensation, and thus the less tendency to draw back from it. I am not talking about injury here; that will be discussed in a later chapter. Injury to the tissues and bones is again information that says, "Pay attention here!" Yet, even with injury, a person with a strong ability to control the mind will feel less pain; like my friend who can have his teeth filled at the dentist without novocaine. (Believe me, that is admirable! I practically need novocaine to walk *into* the dentist's office, never mind to get my teeth filled.)

I have noticed that whenever things get going too fast, and there is too much physical or mental input to work with, I begin to tense up and withdraw. Some of my Rolfing sessions were quite painful, but I was so interested in change, and felt so wonderful afterward, that I was willing to work with it. I remember learning to go right into the sensation, focus my awareness "underneath" the sensation, and watch it as a sensation. It took a lot of attention and concentration, but it worked. I was fascinated to feel exactly how I was holding on, when before I had no idea I was holding at all.

As we've noted before, Dr. Rolf said that Rolfing is more about education than about the medical amelioration of symptoms. Learning about how to work with strong sensation is one of the things I am attempting to teach my clients during the Rolfing process. It has been and continues to be a wonderful challenge for me (someone who has been so afraid of pain) to work with my

The degree to which you respond, modulate, and discriminate non-painful stimuli determines how well you can modulate painful sensation.

— IDA P. ROLF

clients on their issues of pain and fear. I learn every day from my clients what it means to face and deal with holding on to old trauma. In the course of our work together, when we get to difficult areas, I sometimes tell my client that this process is like throwing up. No one would sign up for it; it's no fun to do; but afterward you feel so much better.

I end this chapter with this photograph of Dr. Rolf Rolfing a baby (Figure 7.1) to remind you that there are also many enjoyable parts to a Rolfing session.

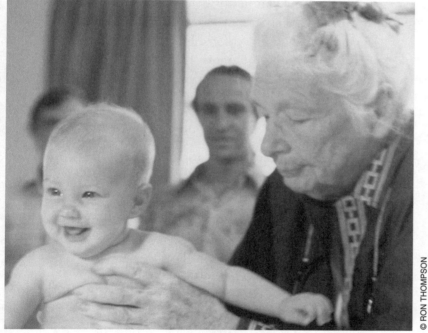

Pleasure is resilience to stimulus – pain is resistance to stimulus.
— IDA P. ROLF

Figure 7.1
Ida P. Rolf, "Rolfing Baby"

TERENCE'S STORY

Terence is a businessman. I did not do his Rolfing, but ran into his story in the course of a business meeting with him. I know and respect his Rolfer, Patricia Stepan, and found his story a fascinating illustration of the cumulative effect of releasing an old pattern that is held in the flesh.

I'd gone through a divorce in the middle 1980s that was extremely painful for both parties and I wanted to make the best use of the experience so that the next time I had a relationship this didn't happen. I was going through therapy – post divorce therapy – sometimes once and twice a week, just to track what was going on with me. The therapist suggested that I try some alternative ways of looking at how I was attempting to deal with uncovering issues in my life. At that time there was a suspicion that something was going on in my family history that nobody had previously uncovered. In conversation with people I learned that Rolfing was really radical; that there was something cutting edge about it, but that you really needed to make the leap.

At that point I really *was* making the leap – by moving into dealing with issues in my life directly. I even had a timeframe that required that I really *get with it*, as opposed to sitting back and intellectualizing about it. Somebody told me about this Rolfer, a woman named Patricia Stepan, and said she was really very good. So I called her up and off we went.

The Rolfing process actually took two years because I had a false start for the first year. I went through probably about sixty or seventy percent of the cycle and then didn't go back, because I kept stretching out the meetings longer and longer; there's a period, a frequency you have to maintain, and I just couldn't do it because I felt it was too painful. I thought it was painful in the body sense – like physical pain – and actually what I learned the second time around was that I was really avoiding the real emotional pain that I literally was carrying in the cells of my body. Although at that time I didn't believe any of that stuff was true. I've learned since that's what really happens. So, I came back the next year and actually went through the whole series, which was nice.

Rolfing made me realize that my body speaks to me in truth…my psychology can hide things and manipulate things, but my body doesn't. One of the overwhelming introductions for me to that was the example of…[my Rolfer] scanning my body with her hand and…intuitively with her finger pressing a point in my body and my body starting to react to whatever was stored there. At that time I didn't believe any of that. But that's what happened. By her doing that, she started a whole chain of emotional movement in me and she began to work with that. As the Rolfing session progressed she would allow that to emerge and work with that energy. To me it was surprising and kind of overwhelming because of the reaction I had. The strength of it was

Pain is a great motivator. It gets our attention and tells us that what we are doing may no longer be working. When something hurts badly enough, we are often more willing to make changes.
– CHRISTINA SELL, YOGA FROM THE INSIDE OUT, 29.

unexpected and every time it came up, for quite awhile, it was stronger and stronger until the point where sometimes I was actually manifesting my pain of being a five year old.

People could say, "Well, this is weird," but the proof of it is that I went through it and I can't deny what I experienced. Patricia was a great guide for that, so I did fully complete the second series of ten sessions.

During the time he was getting this round of Rolfing, Terence attended an intensive psychological growth workshop during which he had a major breakthrough in self-understanding. As he puts it,

> I had a huge opening in my life that revealed one of the hang-ups that was emerging through my Rolfer's work. I was so present. I tie this back to Rolfing.
>
> What was showing up in my body totally bypassed my psychological stuff and my emotional stuff. All of a sudden I had this perspective about one of the major issues in my life that I was hiding from; it had been imbedded in my body energetically, and hidden away in my mind psychologically just to protect myself.
>
> After this shift, one thing after the next *worked* in my life, over the course of two and a half years. (And that's pretty quick to make these huge leaps.) I attribute that to my Rolfing.

I'm still working on what I learned, and my whole life now is about moving forward and challenging myself with where I'm hanging out – where I'm trying to hide. I figure my body just came alive.

During this two-year process of unfolding, Terence met his future wife! Certainly there can be no scientific claim that getting Rolfed will bring you to your future mate, but the opening and reorganization of structure does have some interesting results as clients have indicated.

Endnotes, Chapter 7

[1] Watson, Craig, M.D., Ph.D. *Basic Human Neuroanatomy: An Introductory Atlas second edition*. Boston, Massachusetts: Little, Brown and Company, 1977,13.

[2] Ganong, William F., M.D. *Review of Medical Physiology 7th Edition*. Los Altos, California: Lange Medical Publications, 1975, 76.

[3] Ibid., 77.

[4] Pert, Candace B., Ph. D. *The Molecules of Emotion: Why You Feel the Way You Feel*. New York, N.Y.: Scribner, 1997, 141.

[5] Hutchins, Emmett. Interview. Kauai, Hawaii. June 9, 2004.

[6] Wing, Tom. Interview. Olympia, Washington. March 25, 2004.

Part IV
The Training

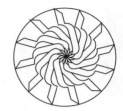

8
What Does It Take to Become a Rolfer?

Back in 1977 when I decided to train as a Rolfer, I had to be twenty-five years old (no problem with that!), have a college degree or other equivalent life experience, have a degree from a massage school (which gave me a license to touch a body), and a background in anatomy, physiology and kinesiology. I had to have been Rolfed, had a number of Rolf Movement sessions, and have enough experience and knowledge in psychology to be aware of transference and countertransference, as well as mature enough to deal with clients when their issues came up during a session. I had to be large enough, in size and weight, with a strong joint structure. In those days I had to send a photograph of myself in underwear, as well as a photograph of my hand, palm up with a quarter in it. I had to have the recommendation of my Rolfer, and to have written a paper for the Rolf Institute that answered certain questions demonstrating my knowledge of anatomy and my experience of having been Rolfed.

Then came the notorious selection interview. For me it was upstairs in the old Pearl Street dance studio in Boulder, where Rolf classes were held at that time. I'm not usually afraid of interviews because all I have to do is respond to questions, not give a speech. So I went into the interview pretty relaxed, but also a bit spaced out, as I was newly with my spiritual teacher and on a vegetarian diet and obnoxiously self righteous about having a teacher.

Those of us who had flown in from various places were waiting our turn in a little anteroom. Occasionally someone would come out of the interview room in tears, having not been accepted or been told to wait. Others would come out glowing and happy. The tension was acute! When it was my turn, I entered the room and found an empty chair facing eight men who sat in a semicircle around it. I knew this was no ordinary interview. These people could *see*. There was to be no bullshitting here!

I can't remember all the questions I was asked, but the main one was why did I want to become a Rolfer. I didn't really know the answer to that question at the time, because my own process had not caught up yet with the unfolding of events that had led me there. Then the committee members looked at the structure of my hands and came up and tested the joints of my fingers. Then I was sent out while they discussed me. Finally, I was called back in…and accepted. What a relief!

My Rolf Training, 1977

The first part of the training was called the Auditor Phase: six weeks of sitting in class watching the teachers (Jan Sultan, with Tom Wing as the assistant) and the practitioners take three people through the Ten Sessions of Rolfing. The whole experience was Zen-like, as I look back on it. It was basically about learning to see – not in a didactic left-brained way, but from a deep, organic, physical-intuitive place. After hanging out in the energy of that Rolfing classroom, being in the field of bodies and people changing, of structures shifting and coming into line, our sight began to slowly deepen. We had to learn to trust what we saw, no matter how strange or slight.

What was challenging throughout this phase was that we were not allowed to touch anyone or do any manipulation for the full six weeks. Our task was just to be present, hang out with awareness, not fall asleep, ask our teachers for information, and watch the teacher's demos carefully. Such observation demanded tremendous patience and acceptance. We watched the unfolding of the Ten Sessions; we noted typical changes that might happen after working in a particular area, and what kinds of reactions the clients might have. We learned to discriminate between our own feelings and those of the clients who were releasing toxins and emotions.

After certain sessions in this training period we might notice that we were feeling irritable or tired. Then we would remember that a client had released a lot of anger, or that there were subtle undertones of clients' emotions hanging out just beneath the surface of openly conscious awareness. We watched how the teachers handled the situation when clients or practitioners had emotional releases. If someone was not balanced at the end of a session, or felt spacey or ungrounded, we observed how the teachers got them present, grounded and balanced. We had to let go of the endless desire to measure up to a particular standard, a grade, or the question "How am I doing?" Such auditing was the antithesis of our normal scholastic experiences of the past. We just got what we got, how we got it, in our own system.

The next phase, called Practitioner training, was preceded by one week of anatomy as it pertains to the sessions, and one week of Rolf Movement Education. We would study the anatomy of each particular session and palpate (explore by touching) on each other. There had to be major cooperation as a group (there were six practitioners) as we practiced on each other to find and feel particular muscles. It could get pretty annoying to have someone

Hold your hands out gently. Ask others to do the same. See how different each person looks. Each person has their own unique and natural beauty. Use this natural beauty when you dance. Respect your individuality.

– ARTEMIS MOURAT

poking around trying to find your piriformis or psoas muscle, and we were all glad we were going to be Rolfed in the approaching class.

During the second preliminary week we looked at movement and its application to Rolfing: What was optimal movement in walking, sitting, and general tasks. We had watched a lot of actual Rolfing in the previous Auditor phase, and now we were to consider some of the movement goals to look for in each of the Ten Sessions.

The first day of Practitioner Training dawned at last, with Emmett Hutchins as my teacher and Tom Wing as the assistant. We had already chosen our class partners, an often challenging and emotional process with only six people. This partner would be the person, like it or not, with whom we were going to make the journey through the basic Ten Sessions.

On Day One we listened to Emmett's lecture on the first hour of the Rolfing sessions; watched him do the first hour work on a model; received the first hour from our class partner; and gave the first hour to our class partner. The second day followed the same pattern, except that we Rolfed our first model. The third day we gave each other the second hour; the fourth day we gave our model the second hour...and so on, in this pattern, through the remaining weeks of class. We were learning on all modes – seeing, touching, being touched, and hearing. We were going through the Ten-Session process ourselves, and at the same time taking two models and our class partner through that series. Wonderfully intense and totally absorbing, this six weeks provided one of the best educational experiences of my life.

At the end of the training I was a Certified Rolfer, and went home to Tucson, Arizona, to establish a practice. The training I had received allowed me to work safely and effectively with clients as I continued to learn the underlying principles embedded in the

In the auditing stage, we were not allowed to touch. Just look...until we finally saw....Ida was asked a lot why she set up the auditing in that way. She would give one of her sighs, roll her eyes, and then say she hadn't found a better way to change people's way of looking and seeing differently. She was trying to teach us to see things in relationship (among other things) and not the linear way that we had been taught.

– BEVERLY SILVERMAN, REMEMBERING IDA ROLF, 92.

Ten-Session Series, Dr. Rolf's "Recipe." I was on my way to learning how to be a chef and not a cook.

Training in the 21st Century

Today the training to become a Rolfer has shifted somewhat. Over the years, prospective Rolfers began coming with more sophisticated background in bodywork, many having been massage therapists, cranio-sacral therapists, and having had experience in other fields of bodywork. At the Rolf Institute school, the Auditor Phase was changed so that it involved the practitioners Rolfing each other without models. In the second phase the practitioners took three models through the Ten-Session Series.

The Guild for Structural Integration maintains the original auditing pattern of watching Rolfing, although it has added other learning activities as well. Both schools take their trainings of future Rolfers seriously even though each reflects a different focus on the breadth and scope of Rolfing.

In the catalog of information on trainings in Structural Integration, GSI states its mission as follows:

1. Structural Integration is a method and a philosophy of personal growth and integrity.
2. The vertical line is our fundamental concept. The physical and psychological embodiment of the vertical line is a way of BEING in the physical world. It forms a basis for personal growth and integrity.
3. The teaching of Structural Integration is transmitted through a form called the "Recipe." The "Recipe is the tradition, the foundation, the essence of Dr. Ida Rolf's teachings.[1]

The Guild for Structural Integration can be reached at:
3107 28th St.
Boulder, CO 80301
800-447-0150
E-MAIL: GSI@rolfguild.org
Web: http:/www.rolfguild.org

The Rolf Institute of Structural Integration states their purpose in their training catalog as follows:

The purpose of the Rolf Institute of Structural Integration is to bring the benefits of Rolfing to the world. This goal is accomplished through providing a quality training program in Rolfing structural integration, certifying Rolfing practitioners and providing them with continuing education, promoting research and educating the public about the value of Rolfing.[2]

The Rolf Institute can be reached at:
5055 Chaparral Ct. Suite 103
Boulder, CO 80301
800-803-1952
E-mail: admissions@rolf.org
http: www.rolf.org

Endnotes, Chapter 8

[1] *Guild for Structural Integration: General Information and Training Programs 2001-2005*. Boulder, Colorado: Guild for Structural Integration, 2001, 2.
[2] *Rolf Institute Educational Catalog 2003-2004*. Boulder, Colorado: Rolf Institute of Structural Integration, 2003, 2.

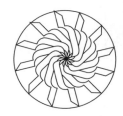

9
Learning To See

Learning to see structure, patterns, energy fields and structural patterns in movement are all keys to doing good Rolfing. You can't change what you can't see just as you can't heal a wound you don't know you have. A Rolfer must learn to see relationships and be able to move back and forth between seeing specific structural patterns and how these patterns relate to each other, and seeing how specific structural components relate to the whole being. As I learned in my first class of auditing with Jan Sultan and Tom Wing, seeing was not just something done with the eyes. As Carlos Castaneda put it, "...I had rallied some knowledge I was not aware of. If that was called seeing, the logical conclusion for my intellect would be to say that seeing is a bodily knowledge."[1]

Part of learning to see is noticing one's own judgments and habit patterns, and beginning to feel the difference between looking and seeing. For me, looking has no depth. It's as though my eyes bounce off the object at which I am looking. Seeing penetrates in a deep and gentle way into what I am observing. My eyes and body become soft, relaxed and open. It is as though the information comes into my being and I *receive* sight through my eyes

Sight is touch at a distance.

– IDA P. ROLF

and body. In contrast to this, looking feels like reaching out with the eyes and grabbing information. With looking there is more of a tendency to behold the object through the lens of my mind and all its preconceived notions. Seeing is receiving what the thing observed has to give to me, so real resonance and subtle communication must be established.

In seeing there is the seer and the seen, and to be truly seen by one who knows how to see deeply can be a profound experience. Tom Wing relates here his experience of being seen by Dr. Rolf:

Just before the end of that class [his Rolfing auditor class] a thing happened that was important to me. Occasionally, when I would be sitting there watching the class, I'd feel her [Dr. Rolf's] gaze on me. You *could* feel it – she had eyes like an eagle, you know. If she turned her attention to you, you knew it. Even if you didn't see it, you could feel it. There would be times when I could feel her looking at me and I would stare straight ahead. I wasn't going to let her know that I knew she was looking. I wasn't going to look at her, for sure. Then, just before the…class ended, I was sitting there minding my own business again and I felt her doing that. I just sort of lost it. It was like one time too many and I thought, *well to hell with it!* I turned my head and she was looking at me and she locked her eyes on my eyes. My gosh! My autonomic nervous system went crazy. I went hot, I went cold, I broke into a sweat, chills and shivers, you know, the whole works…The whole autonomic system just freaked out at being locked in Ida's gaze. There was a sense that she was looking into the deepest part of me; that I was being totally, absolutely, without any reservation whatsoever, being seen; that she saw me. I mean like she knew what I had for breakfast on the morning of my fifth birthday, and that kind of stuff. Then, when

she finished, it felt O.K. As soon as she saw everything
there was to see, she just turned her head away, and it was-
n't a turning from. She just turned her attention to something else.

What I realized was that I felt for the first time in my
life something that I had yearned for all my life and never
[knew] it, which was that I had been totally and absolutely seen by somebody without judgment, just accepted. It
was just a scanning to see *what was* and she had done that.
It was a great gift, an incredible gift, to be seen like that.[2]

Models for Seeing

It is often helpful to use certain abstractions as a way to teach
oneself a broader range of ways to see. One of the simplest and
most basic models is the "blocks model" depicted in the Rolf Logo
shown in Figure 9.1. Granted, it is a static model and does not
involve movement, but it is easy to see that there are sets of relationships that depend on each other. Any child knows from experience that if you are using blocks you must have a good base of
support to build a tower that won't fall over. Even from this simple diagram one can see that problems in the neck and shoulders
may often come from an imbalance in the pelvis and legs.

There are many other models that Rolfers may use to enhance
their seeing of structure. Emmett Hutchins used one that he called
a "functional archetype of a two-way operator." This involves considering the relationship between two opposing forces. A simple
example would be wringing out a wash cloth. Each end of the
cloth is moved in opposition, with one rotational force moving
clockwise and one moving counterclockwise. To release the
"wring" in the middle, one needs to work at either end. To translate this example into the body: wherever there is shortness and

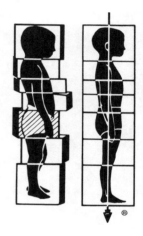

Figure 9.1
The Rolf Logo

lack of movement in one place, there will usually be another place of holding that matches.

I could have a client lying on his back and work with the relationship of the heel to the top of the fibula, while intending to match these two pieces with a central line going through the leg. Emmett would call this abstraction a "trinity," where there is a unifying principle that brings the polar opposites together.[3] Once you find this central principle, which in Rolfing is the Line, you are no longer locked in an oppositional battle.

In my practitioner class with Emmett Hutchins and Tom Wing we were encouraged to imagine and believe that the body could change in any way that we could see, whether it made sense anatomically or not. I was often amazed that when I would use these abstractions both to see and work, the body *did* change in ways I would have never imagined possible.

An analytical person is good at asking the right questions in the right order to come to a conclusion. A simple example of this might be to ask why is the right shoulder on a client higher than on the left. One might see then that the ribcage on the left side is dropped and the scapula has less support. Why are the left ribs dropped? One might then see that there is a lateral curvature that has caused the vertebrae to rotate with the spinous processes back to the right, and a side bending of the vertebral bodies to the left, and so on. Then one would look at this pattern from the front, side and back, continuing to ask questions. Quite an intricate amount of detail can be gathered with this method. The trick is to keep this detail in mind as you work and still be able step back now and then to look at the whole. Detailed knowledge of anatomy is a must for Rolfers, but it can also get in the way if one becomes too linear and dependent upon it. This anonymous quote found in my class notes says it well: "Show a man too many camel bones and show them to him too often and he will not be able to recognize a camel when he sees one."

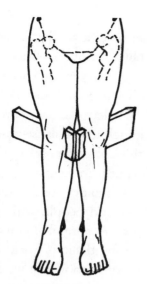

Figure 9.2a
"X legs" (valgus variation): laterally rotated femurs, commonly called
"knock-kneed"

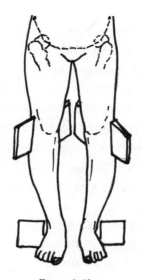

Figure 9.2b
"O legs" (varus variation): medially
rotated femurs, commonly called
"bow-legged"

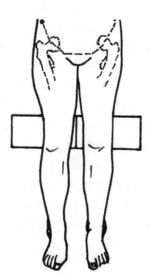

Figure 9.2c
Normally aligned legs

Other Rolfers have developed other specific models – such as the X and O leg model first introduced by Jan Sultan.[4] Briefly, this model evolves from the fact that there are two general patterns of the femur that set up other patterns in the legs and feet. A laterally rotated femur is considered an X or valgus variation on normal. In this pattern the person looks knock-kneed as is shown in Figure 9.2a (see previous page). I see this pattern most often in a more soft body, or a more *kapha* type to put it in Ayurvedic terms. A medially rotated femur is an O or varus variation, as is shown in Figure 9.2b. I see this often in athletes and people with more mesomorphic and ectomorphic body types. A normal alignment is shown in Figure 9.2c. The places where the tissue is stuck, overworked and built up is due to the variation in how the weight is transmitted through the thigh and leg in each of these patterns. Being able to recognize such variations is helpful in strategizing a session, as each pattern clearly demands work in areas specific to that pattern.

Robert Schleip, in his articles from "Talking to Fascia," has also proposed an interesting neurobiological model for describing habitual body patterns that often develop during infancy.

This model looks at two primary reaction patterns that are sometimes called reflexes: the "Landau Reflex" as a basis for a chronic shortening of most genetic extensor muscles and the "Startle Reflex" as a basis for chronic shortening of most genetic flexor muscles. It is suggested that the two mentioned reaction patterns involving those two opposing sets of muscles – the genetic extensors and the genetic flexors – can be understood as important forces influencing adult human structures.[5]

For some people the muscular pattern of the startle reflex becomes a dominant feature in their general posture and movement

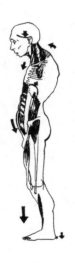

Figure 9.3
Flexors overused
From Emotional Anatomy:
The Structure of
Experience *by Stanley
Keleman.*
Used with permission.

(*see* Figure 9.3). Moshe Feldenkrais, in his book *The Body and Mature Behavior*, called attention to the fact that in all negative emotion the flexors of the body contract.[6] There is plenty of emotional experience that is negative floating around on Planet Earth during anyone's development in life. Consider the cycle this can set up with a constant underlying tension, the general feeling of anxiety and depression that accompanies such a physical pattern.

The opposite pattern based on the Landau reflex is depicted in the typical military style posture shown in Figure 9.4, which shortens the extensors of the body. The accompanying feeling here is the readiness to fight, to "take it on the chin," so to speak. The key in Rolfing, as well as in seeing how to proceed in a session, is to help people to become free of rigid patterns of any kind that limit options. Ideally one could be prepared to run or fight when appropriate and not have to waste energy in a constant pattern of expectancy. Interestingly, a body stance or way of moving sends out a message to others. A person who stands and moves in the posture of a victim tends to get picked on. A person all puffed up and rigid who looks ready to fight at any minute will often attract personal confrontations.

Another fascinating place to look for habit patterns in structure is the carriage of the arms. In your nearest high school or mall you will find wonderful examples of what I call "attitude walks" that involve a particular expression of the arms. When the elbows are carried close to the body and behind the lumbodorsal hinge, and the palms turned outward, the feeling that one receives from that person is a giving away of her own personal power. The solar plexus is totally exposed and there is no sense of center, no principle of verticality. The person is not aware of or in control of her own center. Another common pattern is the "tough guy." The arms are rotated inward and carried a bit away from the body. The feeling here is one of unavailability and a lack of resilience. The arms are protecting the heart and ready for defense.

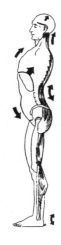

Figure 9.4
Extensors overused
From Emotional Anatomy:
The Structure of
Experience *by Stanley
Keleman.*
Used with permission.

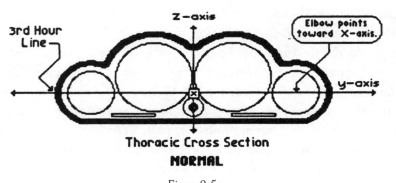

Figure 9.5a

Cross section of a balanced shoulder girdle, viewed from the top

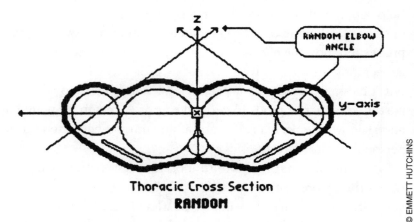

Figure 9.5 b

Cross section of shoulder girdle showing overdevelopment of the muscles that rotate the humerus medially, viewed from the top

Arms reflect a tremendous amount of what is happening in the neck, head and ribcage. Dr. Rolf would emphasize that if the arms and shoulder girdle were balanced, the elbows would be able to move directly to the side without pulling the humerus forward toward the midline. Computer drawings developed by Emmett

Hutchins show a cross section of the shoulder girdle viewed from the top. Figure 9.5a shows a balanced shoulder girdle and Figure 9.5b shows an overdevelopment of the muscles that rotate the humerus medially. Seen from the front, the fascial line that runs from the thumb up the medial side of the arm to the clavicle and front of the neck should have enough length to accommodate that fascial line that runs from the little finger through the lateral side of the arm and across the shoulder blade to the back of the neck.

Head carriage and eye position probably show the most expression. With a partner try the following eye and head positions, and notice what you feel both in yourself and in your partner as you face each other:

- Head lowered and eyes up.
- Head raised with eyes looking down the nose.
- Head rigidly straight and eyes staring straight.
- Head relaxed and even with eyes softly looking straight.
- Eyes should shine out like headlights from the back of the head as shown in Figure 9.6.

The illustrations and discussions here are by necessity two dimensional and static due to the verbal medium, and might suggest that there is one ideal template of perfect structure toward which we Rolfers are attempting to herd everyone. If there was any static template it would be one of neutrality – the neutrality that is present before movement. To me the keys are resilience, adaptability and expression. How can Jane Smith best express the best Jane Smith who might be from a particular class, country, race, body type or size? How can she have all the options possible for her own movement, expression and growth? If I as a Rolfer can aid Jane Smith, my hypothetical client, to release patterns that restrict her and cause her pain, and help her to find her own sense

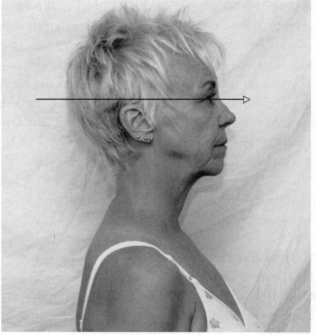

Figure 9.6
Aligned head and eyes

of "up" from within her own center as she moves forward with more options and choices in her life, and if we can do this together, this would be a great Ten-Session Series for us both!

There are far more models for seeing and ways to see than can be covered by the scope of this book. However, some general things that I might look for as I watch the client walk or do small movements, such as little knee bends or raising the arms up over the head or out to the side, or turning the head from right to left are:

- How does the movement travel through the body?
- Where does it stick or pull on another body part?

- Do I see certain muscles standing out more than others?
- What is the alignment of the legs?
- What is the overall feeling of the movement? Flowing and graceful? Hesitant? Taking a lot of energy?
- I might also get a feeling of the level of energy of the client, his color, skin texture, emotional tone, the energy I feel coming from him.
- Is there a balance between the major weight blocks of head, shoulders, torso, pelvis, legs, or does for example the chest look much smaller and more immature than the legs and feet?
- Is there someplace in the body where growth seems to have stopped at a certain age?

In a Rolfing class one has plenty of time to sit and go into the space of seeing because the class models and practitioners are prepared to stand and move for quite awhile while the students discuss what they see. In my own private practice I must get a quick hit and see enough to begin the session, as most clients are a bit self conscious standing in front of someone in their underwear! Later, as I begin to work and interact with the client, I get more information along the way. How do they walk into the room each week? What does their emotional and physical energy feel like today? What do they choose to tell me when I ask them how they are doing? I feel that people inherently want to be seen. Tom Wing put it well when he noticed this pattern over the hours of watching Rolfing in his auditor's class. "And it felt like, 'See me. Please see me, but don't look. Don't look.' And there was that back and forth, that desire to be seen but an aversion to being looked at. And I think that part of what draws people to Rolfing is an unconscious perception that Rolfers are people who see you." [7]

Yes, Rolfers should be people who see you.

Over the years your bodies become walking autobiographies, telling friends and strangers alike of the minor and major stresses of your lives.

– MARILYN FERGUSON

MARY'S STORY

After receiving the basic Ten Series of Rolfing, Mary told her story:

I am a musician and a painter. Before I began my Rolfing sessions I was having problems with my hands. My index finger on the left hand was feeling weak and I had to cancel a performance due to my inability to practice. Also, my hands were both tingling and going numb at night. At the end of each day after housework, practicing and painting, the bones in my hands were so sore that often I could not get to sleep. The work I received from my Rolfer has allowed me to revive my practice schedule and has improved my playing in general. My hands no longer fall asleep at night and also the soreness at the end of the day is gone. I found as I was receiving the work that no matter what muscles were being worked, my gut began to relax and so far the effect has remained. My digestion is vastly improved and also my breathing has deepened to levels I have never experienced before. My diaphragm freely expands and contracts without any effort on my part. This is a most wonderful effect as I have had many physical problems as a result of childhood sexual abuse. I do believe I have been given a second chance to enjoy my physical body at age forty-eight.

Endnotes, Chapter 9

[1] Castaneda, Carlos. *The Eagle's Gift*. New York, New York: Simon and Schuster, Inc., 1981, 37.

[2] Wing, Tom. Interview. March 25, 2004.

[3] Ibid.

[4] Sultan, Jan. Rolf class notes.

[5] Schleip, Robert. "Talking to Fascia – Changing the Brain: A Collection of Articles on Rolfing and the Nero-Myofascial Net. Reprinted from *Rolf Lines*. Boulder, Colorado: The Rolf Institute, October, 1993, 3.

[6] Feldenkrais, Moshe. *The Body and Mature Behavior: A Study of Anxiety, Sex, Gravitation and Learning*. New York, N.Y.: International Universities Press, 1950.

[7] Wing, Tom. Interview March 25, 2004.

Part V
The Special Considerations

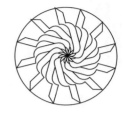

10
Special Considerations in Rolfing

Rolfing Babies, Children and Teenagers

It is a gift to Rolf children – a gift to their future development and a gift to the Rolfer to be involved in their growth. For a sensitive Rolfer who is familiar and comfortable with babies, a child's Rolfing could begin as early as is acceptable to both baby and mother. When I was visiting Emmett Hutchins in Kauai he had some photos of a tiny premature baby he had worked with, the youngest in his thirty-five years of practice as a Rolfer. She was born three months premature and only weighed one-and-one-half pounds. When Emmett worked with her she had gained a bit and was up to four pounds. This infant had feeding tubes and breathing tubes attached to her body that were restricting her shoulder girdle and spine. On such a tiny child all one needs is barely a touch with clear intention. Emmett worked to lengthen her spine and free her shoulder girdle and those present could see the change in her. The principles of Rolfing can work in a large variety of situations and the level of touch can be adjusted to suit the newborn or the armored football player.

Usually a baby's mother will have noticed a particular pattern in her infant, such always reaching with the same hand, or only turning the head one way, or kicking more with one leg than the other. A gentle, focused ten or fifteen minutes of work can encourage a child to move that limb that was restricted in utero or stressed during the birth process. Just a small adjustment and the child is assisted to grow in a more balanced way.

My intention is always to include the child in the process, so I explain directly to him or her briefly what I am going to do. Little children and babies who are not yet talking will still feel the intention and respond. Figure 10.1, a photo of Dr. Rolf Rolfing a baby, shows a deep level of communication between the two. Most children really take to being Rolfed, as they intuitively know it is going to help them. Some just come in and get up on the table like

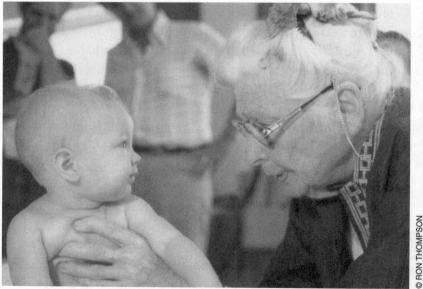

© RON THOMPSON

Figure 10.1
Ida P. Rolf, "Eye to Eye"

they are old hands; others like something to play with while I am working with them.

With the crawlers and toddlers, I often engage them on the floor where they can move around a bit. One five year old with whom I worked quite extensively loved coming to get Rolfed so much that she would Rolf her dolls and offer to Rolf any guest that would show up at her house. During her sessions I would let her play with a little plastic skeleton that I had on hand to show people a bit about structure. Even at that young age she was interested in how the body worked and would ask questions. She called it "Skeletor" and happily played with it while I Rolfed her. Whenever she felt that she needed a Rolfing session she would let her mother know.

Short, focused sessions – from ten minutes to half an hour – seem to work best with young children and babies; and they clearly let you know when they have had enough! Usually I do not give children a formal Ten-Session Series until they are ten or twelve years old. A few small adjustments here and there in a child, or more focused work if there is a specific developmental problem, is generally enough to send them growing toward a new level of integration and alignment.

As young children have not yet developed their deep intrinsic muscles, I don't ask them to do some of the finer movements that I might ask of adults during Rolfing. Children are growing outward, developing their egos and sense of "me," so I don't ask them to go inward. They are more interested in being able to run better, kick the ball further, or perhaps stand a little straighter.

When a child is just beginning to enter puberty it is a time to be particularly sensitive to his or her growth process. Rolfing can make some profound changes in the structure. Some young teens are already having so many hormonal and bodily changes that they are a bit resistant to having more changes with the Rolfing. However, most young people at this age really enjoy the Rolfing as

I am convinced that life in a physical body is meant to be an ecstatic experience.

– SHAKTI GAWAIN

it helps them to transition more easily through puberty and gives them a positive feeling about their developing bodies. Along these lines, sometimes it is better for the pre-teen to be Rolfed by some-one of the same sex; although this is not always an issue. The child or adolescent should know ahead of time that they are going to be Rolfed in their underwear or bathing suit. If there is a particular issue over getting undressed I will sometimes begin to Rolf them in their T-shirts or shorts. The most important consideration is that they feel comfortable. Each teen is different, of course, and so listening to their experience of the Rolfing and feeling out where they are in the process is vital. I make sure in the initial interview with the parent and child that Rolfing is something that the teen wants to do.

Most of the time a parent is present during the Rolfing session, until both parent and child feel comfortable with the Rolfer and the process. As the child grows older, having the parent leave and run errands during the Rolfing session allows me to establish a deeper rapport with the young person. Some teens in particular are more open *without* the parent around. Occasionally the dynamics between parent and child will curtail my relationship to the child; and, some parents will engage me in such an interesting way that I have to be careful not to lose focus on the child.

Birth trauma, accidents, injuries, illness and abuse all leave their mark in the growing child's physical and emotional structure. To release and realign the tissues early in the child's life, before they get set in the fascia, will make a big difference in how the child develops later on. (*See* Figure 10.2)

Older Folks

My mother received her first Ten-Session Series of Rolfing when she was in her early seventies, and loved it. She said it helped her general balance and gave her more confidence in her walking

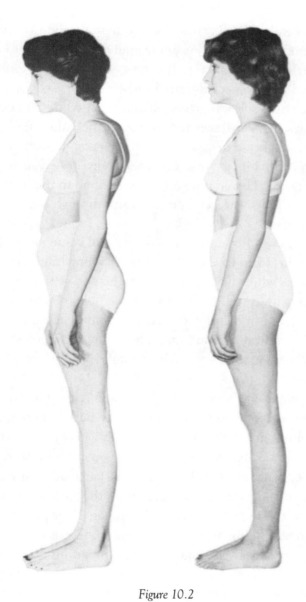

Figure 10.2

Before one session   *After ten sessions*

"Chris" before and after, from The Promise of Rolfing Children *by Robert Toporek.*

Used with permission.

and tennis. I Rolfed her until she was in her late eighties, and she always responded positively. As her overall energy grew less I needed to make the sessions shorter, however, so as not to overtire her. I also needed to be especially careful when she first got up off the table to make sure she was grounded and oriented in her body.

The oldest person I ever took through the basic Ten-Session Series was an eighty-four-year-old man. His granddaughter would bring him in, help him get undressed and then dressed again at the end of the session. He did not seem present at all in the beginning, and I felt like I was energetically shouting through a megaphone to a distant planet, "*Hello! Hello!* Is anyone home?" As we went along in the Series he started to wake up and come alive again. I kept turning his focus toward his body and asking him to make little movements while I was working. By the end of the Ten Series he was talking away, telling stories. He was able to come in to the session unassisted, and undress and dress by himself. He stood a little taller and moved a little more freely. The most powerful part was that he seemed to have decided to wake up and live what was left of his life.

Older people are somewhat like children in that they may need shorter sessions and a lighter touch, but beyond that the goals of Rolfing may be somewhat different. People near the last third or fourth of their lives need to stay open and resilient. For older people, being grounded in the feet is particularly important. During the death process the feeling leaves the feet first and works its way up to the heart and head. Getting an older person to feel his feet, and reminding him to be aware of his feet as he walks, will help him a great deal with balance. An important goal of many older folks is to be able to stay functioning relatively pain free. Gravity pulls strongly on anything that is out of line, such as an overly curved back or a forward-reaching head. Getting more length, space, and organization in any body at any age will give a person a real physical and psychological lift.

I get up. I walk. I fall down. Meanwhile, I keep dancing.

— HILLEL

Often, older people have had surgery. Sometimes there are circulatory problems, such as varicose veins. Their skin may be thin and sensitive. For these and other reasons special care needs to be taken. Anyone being Rolfed should have enough energy and basic good health to be able to receive and assimilate the work. The connective tissue should have a generally healthy feel, and no acute inflammatory pathology should be present. Careful neck and spine work helps to give space to the vital nerve and blood vessel pathways to the head, allowing for better functioning. Work around the ribcage and diaphragm keeps the breathing full, which in turn energizes the whole body.

In working with people in their seventies and eighties, I notice how important their attitude is. Oldsters who are generally positive and open make changes equally as dramatic as younger folks in their twenties and thirties. How rewarding for anyone to feel like she could actually change her structure late in life! As far as I'm concerned, we can always keep heading for "vertical," right up until the time we eventually end up horizontal for good.

Contraindications for Rolfing

Rolfing is not meant to cure illness or deal with immediate, acute injuries. It should not be used as a substitute for appropriate medical treatment. If you get run over by a bus, you need a doctor not a Rolfer! After the doctor handles the acute situation, *then* you get Rolfed.

It is inadvisable to Rolf someone when they are in the acute or inflammatory stages of a systemic illness. If someone is running a fever, I tell them to wait until the temperature is normal before coming for Rolfing. If an injury is inflamed, red and swollen I do not work directly in that area. If a client has had surgery, especially abdominal surgery, the tissues need to be completely healed before working directly on them.

We are not victims of aging, sickness, and death. These are part of the scenery, not the seer, who is immune to any form of change.
— DEEPAK CHOPRA M.D., AGELESS BODY TIMELESS MIND, 36.

Although Dr. Rolf would take on people with intense pathology, it was usually *structural* pathology from old injuries or illness; in these cases the immediate, acute situation had already healed. She advised us not to Rolf someone who might die on the Rolfing table!

In the early days we were not to work on anyone with cancer who hadn't been in remission for five years. The reason then was that we were not sure whether the deep work in the tissue would spread the cancer. This may have changed in the ensuing years, as many people with cancer now receive massage with no ill effects. However, I always ask for the client's doctor's permission when Rolfing anyone who has had any recent (within the last five years) surgery for cancer.

Rolfing is mainly geared to work with chronic structural problems. Occasionally, if an acute structural problem, such as a sprained ankle, can be worked on immediately, before the swelling and pain set in, this can bring the proper alignment and space for faster healing. My most graphic example of this was during a hike with a group of women up 14,000-foot Longs Peak in Estes Park, Colorado. Coming back down and just off the summit, one of the women fell and sprained her ankle. After determining that it was most likely not fractured (fortunate because a rescue on this mountain would have taken many hours), I sat her down on a rock and did my best to realign her lower leg and foot so that she was able to walk. We still had a long downhill trek to get back to the campsite at tree line, but she was able, though very slowly, to walk back to this spot, and then on down to the base of the mountain.

If there is a history of deep emotional problems in a client, if he or she is on medication for schizophrenia, psychosis, or bipolar (manic depression), it is necessary to work with the client's psychiatrist or psychologist. I don't usually Rolf people who are psychotic or schizophrenic. (In the next chapter we will consider the subject of trauma.) Again, the rule of thumb is to avoid Rolfing people who are in an acute situation. There are plenty of "normal" neurotics out there who can benefit from Rolfing and I especially love the challenge of helping them to discover their own wisdom as their bodies become more organized.

Once I began working with a young man of about sixteen who had strong mood swings. He loved the Rolfing, but I felt something was "off" about his responses. We got about halfway through the Series when he didn't show up for a session. I called his mother and found out he had been hospitalized for manic depression. No wonder things felt strange! We did not continue the Rolfing as he was too emotionally unstable at the time to be able to assimilate the work. At the time, manic depression, or "bipolar syndrome" as it is now called, was not as well recognized nor treated in the same way. I have since worked very successfully Rolfing a young woman who is bipolar, but she is on medication that stabilizes her swings in mood. As I have a background in psychology and counseling, I can usually recognize when someone needs the assistance of a psychotherapist or psychiatrist for support as they go through the Rolfing.

There are endless surprises that will present themselves to a Rolfer in terms of the physical and emotional pathology of the client. I always listen to my intuition and gut feelings. If there is a lot of fear in me around working with a client, I need to look at that carefully. My approach is to ask enough questions so that I am confidant enough to either go ahead or refer the client to another practitioner.

We are each 100% responsible for all our experiences.
– LOUISE L. HAY, YOU CAN HEAL YOUR LIFE, 5.

Referrals

It is important for Rolfers to establish good relationships with other healing arts practitioners and physicians in the community. Sometimes it is appropriate to refer a client to another practitioner when their problem is beyond the scope of the Rolfer's practice.

The back has become forgotten in our culture. It has been allowed to atrophy, becoming an immovable, wood-like thing "somewhere back there."...When we breathe there is little movement in the back. The back sometimes awakens us out of our forgetfulness by expressing its chronic pain, a pain rooted in the forgetfulness itself.

– DON JOHNSON, THE PROTEAN BODY, 66.

Clients who come in with inflammation of the digestive tract – such as gastritis, ileitis and colitis – need to see a doctor or naturopath to reduce the inflammation first. Later, Rolfing can be helpful by providing more space and better alignment thus assisting in improved functioning of the organs.

If there is an experienced Jin Shin Jyutsu® practitioner or a good acupuncturist in the area I will often refer the client who comes to me in the beginning stages of flu, bronchitis, or pneumonia. If there is a necessity for a doctor's visit or even a hospital stay, Rolfing can be especially helpful during the recovery period after the illness has passed. Illness usually causes the rib angles to drop, the flexor muscles of the body to tighten, and thus the breath becomes shallower. Getting the vertical line back in the body will accelerate healing.

Some Special Cases

The following is a small sample of some of the many "special cases" that have come to me over the years. At times, Rolfing was contraindicated. Overall, however, results have been extremely rewarding for the client.

- A twenty-year-old man had a Harrington rod in his spine for scoliosis. I asked to see x-rays and consulted with his physician. He went through the Ten Series with no problems. However, the change I was able to get in his system was much less than I would ordinarily get because I was unable to work deeply around his spine.
- An eighty-year-old man had an aortic aneurysm. He had already been Rolfed extensively. I consulted with a physician in the Rolf community. I also consulted with and got permission from the man's physician. The

man loves Rolfing and its benefits for him. He continues to receive regular work.

- A child with spina bifida had required several surgeries, one of which was to install a shunt from her brain to her abdominal cavity. She was brought to see me when she was three. This case disturbed me at first. I read the surgery reports, saw the x-rays, located the shunt under my fingers (it was just under the skin and superficial fascia). I consulted with one of my Rolfing teachers and also got the permission of her doctor. This child was fabulous! She loved the Rolfing and benefited a great deal from it. I worked with her for about three years and got to watch her begin to talk, deal with walking in braces, and begin to explore her world.

- A forty-year-old woman had open heart surgery when she was nineteen. She still had the pins in the ribs where her chest was broken open to access the heart. Once I saw the x-rays and could locate where the pins were, I could avoid them when Rolfing her. Even though she was extremely positive about the changes in her body, especially the expanded breathing, she has not yet finished the Ten Series. She ran into some family problems that needed all her attention.

- An overweight eighty-year-old woman had two hip replacements and a seriously misaligned knee. She was referred to me by another Rolfer. I was a bit dubious about the possibility for success, but even though she had to drive an hour each way to get to me, this client was enthusiastic, cooperative and determined. She strongly believed in the work. I consulted her previous Rolfer and looked at the x-rays of her hip replacement surgery. This woman benefited a great deal from the work and she surprised me with the changes we were able to get. She was a good example of the importance of the client's attitude in the process.

- A woman had three surgeries for removal of brain tumors. Other than that she was perfectly healthy, functioning normally, and eager to get Rolfed. I consulted with her doctor and received his O.K. to work with her. This client responded beautifully, and as she was highly aware of her body we were able to learn together. She gave me the courage and go-ahead to work on her head in ways that were effective for her.

- "Joe" was recovering from a stroke and felt that Rolfing might help him to regain some balance in his walking. I consulted with his doctor and got permission to Rolf him. Joe improved greatly in his ability to walk more freely. Later on he had another stroke, and since he had had so much success from the Rolfing after his first stroke, he was back again on my doorstep. Again I consulted his physician. This time the physician said it was O.K. to Rolf Joe, but not to work at all on his neck and head. After consulting with a Rolfer physician I decided against Rolfing Joe anymore, as any changes in the rest of his body could not be integrated through his head and neck. To continue to Rolf him under those circumstances would only place more strain on the very place the doctor did not want me to work. When I explained this to Joe he was extremely disappointed, but he also understood my concerns.

* * *

NORA'S STORY

"Nora" had suffered a severe compound fracture of her left tibia and fibula when she was ski racing in college. With her Rolfing session, received at age thirty-five, she was very aware of her body and a willing client. Today, at sixty-two, she continues to race in the masters program. In the years since the original break, her tibia and fibula have fused together just above her ankle which limited her ability to flex her ankle. What was particularly interesting about her situation was how far we could change her ankle toward the flexion she needs for ski racing without the ankle becoming more painful due to less compensation.

In follow-up Rolfing sessions I would start with her standing and have her slightly bend her knees and ankles and then I would watch for where there was no movement, and where the compensation for this went on up into her hips, back, and eventually neck and head. Then I would work around the ankle, shin, heel and knee until we got a bit of new movement. After that I'd have her lie down and I'd follow the compensatory pattern, releasing that to match the changes we'd gotten below. After several sessions there was a remarkable change in her structure. She was able to move her ankle and knee in a straight line and the whole shape of her lower leg shifted as she came into alignment. We were also able to get just a bit more ankle flexion. Even her physical therapist noticed the change. But the problem was that with the better alignment and freer movement she had more pain. Hmm. We had to consider that there was only so far the ankle could go toward flexion with the fusion of the fibula. However, with a specially fitted ski boot, she has resumed racing without pain.
– Betsy Sise

If my client is a tennis player, one arm and shoulder will be more developed than the other. The Rolfing will keep her from becoming too bound up in her muscles, which in turn will make her less prone to injury. She will become more aware of how she does her swing, and be able to adjust to the least stressful yet most economic movement. Rolfing is meant to make one more resilient and thus more able to change back and forth between forms of movement when needed.
– BETSY SISE

In the end, what keeps Rolfer and client safe is love – unconditional love, or a desire for the highest and best for the client. For me, the spirit of *karma yoga* (doing your best without being attached to the results) is my way of not getting too caught up in results, or in the praise or blame of the client. If I can attempt to do my best, listen to the client, empower her, and really *see* her, usually things work out.

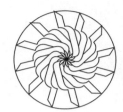

11
Trauma

Early Rolfing and Catharsis

In the late 1960s as Rolfing emerged into the public eye, other modalities were also exploring the mind-body relationship, particularly at Esalen where Dr. Rolf frequently practiced. Some of these modalities, such as Janov's Primal Scream, Lowen's Bioenergetics, and the encounter group movement often involved some catharsis. Pillows were pounded in some encounter groups; screaming and towel pounding were common in Bioenergetics; and of course "the scream" was central to Primal Scream therapy.

I had opportunities to experience these cathartic methods myself. In the mid-1970s, when Alexander Lowen came to Tucson to teach a Bioenergetics workshop, I attended. Part of the class involved taking certain stressful bodily positions such as bending backward over a stool, or lying on one's back with the feet up in the air. A lot of dramatic screaming and crying was going on, but nothing was happening for me. All in all, I found the atmosphere to be pretty crazy. At one point during the session, the instructor came over and pressed hard and painfully on the inside of my thighs. Immediately I became one of the screamers, yelling, "I trusted you and you tricked me."

As I look back on that Bioenergetics class I realize that an old trauma had been re-activated in me, and the same was probably true for many others in that class. The problem, however, was that there was no resolution of this trauma in my psycho-physiological being. The class just went on.

In later years I became involved with studying Gestalt therapy and participated in several groups. True Gestalt therapy as Fritz Perls envisioned it was designed to bring the client to an impasse, and then help him or her through the impasse. Perls' prime dictum was that "awareness is healing." This was aligned with Dr. Rolf's basic ideas of structure determining function. However, as various people began incorporating Gestalt techniques in their groups, many cathartic techniques were used: there was some acting out, some pounding of pillows that were supposed to represent our fathers or mothers; use of *batakas*, a soft fat club that made a satisfying but harmless "whump" when you hit someone. It was all great fun, stimulating, and probably helpful in many ways.

Into this milieu of drama and cathartic modalities came Dr. Rolf, an old Victorian lady, with her vision and technique of Rolfing. She was definitely not into drama and acting out, which might have been why she seemed at times to be so scathing in her assessments of psychotherapy in general. She did, however, have a great respect for Fritz Perls and his Gestalt therapy. Imagine Dr. Rolf at Esalen Institute among the pot-smoking hippies of the 60s and the notorious hot spring baths at Esalen where everyone went nude. She would insist that anyone coming to her for Rolfing wear underwear! When someone would wander in without any clothes, she had spare underwear for them to put on.

At that time Rolfing was something radical – *the* thing to do – and many Rolfees in those years got into the drama of catharsis while they were being Rolfed. There was also an unspoken

Doubt everything. Find your own light.
– GAUTAMA BUDDHA

assumption that Rolfing really wasn't working unless it hurt like hell. Early on, we Rolfers were not familiar with the paradigm that connective tissue was plastic and could change easily. We believed that you had to work extremely hard for change to happen. So, Rolfing became known for being painful, and people loved to tell, often with much exaggeration, their war stories of getting Rolfed. Many of us Rolfers knew little about the physiological and psychological aspects of trauma and so we marched gaily along in our Rolfing, somewhat oblivious to the subtle autonomic responses that signaled the reactivation of a buried trauma. As Rolfing works deep in the connective tissue system, it is bound to bring up trauma residue that has been immobilized and embedded in the fascia.

Dr. Peter Levine and the Physiology of Trauma

In 1990, after having been a Rolfer for twelve years, I ran into Dr. Peter Levine in Boulder, Colorado. Word was going around among the Rolfers that Levine had an exciting new way of healing past trauma, and that it was vital that we as Rolfers have an understanding of the physiology of trauma and how best to recognize and deal with it in our Rolfing sessions. I was fortunate enough to take two workshops with Levine in 1990 and 1991, and the following information is taken from my class notes and from a book Dr. Levine later wrote called *Waking the Tiger: Healing Trauma*.

Levine had long been interested in the mystery behind the large variety of symptoms that would show up in people who had experienced various types of trauma in their lives. He studied medical biophysics as well as animal behavior, and began to notice how animals dealt with trauma. He met Dr. Rolf and became acquainted with Rolfing at Esalen. While at Esalen, he noticed that big cathartic experiences actually made people worse, exacerbating symptoms associated with trauma – such as depression, anxiety, digestive problems and allergies. Levine came to understand from his studies that when people re-enact traumatic events with catharsis, they release endorphins and are then exhilarated. This can result in a perpetual cycle of catharting, reactivating trauma, repressing it again and spiraling back into the physical and emotional symptoms of the original, buried shock of the trauma. Encouraging emotional and even physical catharsis can actually keep a person from getting in touch with his or her body, a necessary factor in the healing of trauma. In the case of pounding the pillow to "release your anger," the experience is more focused on feeling the pounding rather than feeling the often-subtle present-time-sense, deep in the physical body. We are *always* feeling something, but when normal primal feelings are blocked, the secondary emotions of pain, anger, fear, and sadness arise.[1] Distinguishing between emotions and feeling, Paul Oertel notes that: "…emotions can be temporary energistic states based on imbalances and delusions of the mind. Feeling is [the] essential connection to pure uncompromised truth…feeling is a connection to something that is timeless."[2]

The philosophy of suppressing symptoms without considering and evaluating the underlying dynamic is contrary to good health and common sense.

— FRITZ FREDERICK SMITH, M.D., *INNER BRIDGES*, 171.

The Physiology of Trauma

Vital to a basic understanding of trauma in humans is the realization that there are different areas of the brain that each have a different function, yet are interlinked and in communication with each other.

The involuntary and instinctual portions of the human brain and nervous system are virtually identical to those of other mammals and even reptiles. Our brain, often called the triune brain, consists of three integral systems. The three parts are commonly known as the reptilian brain (instinctual), the mammalian or limbic brain (emotional), and the human brain or neo-cortex (rational).[3]

The basic responses to any kind of threat to the system are flight or fight. Every creature has these instinctual mobilizations that orient it toward the source of danger and then toward safety. But, a third response can be seen throughout the animal kingdom, yet is not so immediately apparent in the human. That response is freezing or immobilization and, particularly in the human, dissociation. Dr. Levine describes this in *Waking the Tiger* using the example of a prey animal, such as a rabbit, that has been caught or trapped by the predator. The instinct of the predator is to chase something that is moving. When the rabbit has no means of escape and is unequipped to fight, it goes limp and becomes immobile. This "playing dead" often distracts the predator and the rabbit may then escape. Levine then describes what happens next:

> When it is out of danger, the animal will literally shake off the residual effects of the immobility response and gain full control of its body. It will then return to its normal life as if nothing had happened...Most modern cultures tend to judge this instinctive surrender in the face of overwhelming threat as a weakness tantamount to cowardice. However underneath this judgment lies a deep human fear of immobility. We avoid it because it is a state very similar to death. This avoidance is understandable, but we pay dearly for it. The physiological evidence clearly shows that the ability to go into and come out of this natural response is the key to avoiding the debilitating effects of trauma. It is a gift from the wild.[4]

The key to healing trauma, as Levine states, is in our physiology. As Rolfing is directly working with ordering the physical body, the Rolf practitioner may likely run into the trauma history of his or her client during their sessions.

Tremendous physiological energy is mobilized throughout the body in any perceived danger. Imagine that you are walking home at night and you take a shortcut through an empty lot (stupid move!). You hear an unusual rustle in the bushes nearby and instantly you stop and turn toward the sound, body tensed for flight, heart rate and breathing activated as your body prepares to take action. Before you can move, a man jumps out, grabs you in a viselike grip, and holds a knife to your throat. You struggle but are unable to free yourself. You manage to utter a scream and then collapse and go numb. Luckily a passing patrol car hears your scream, stops, and the attacker runs off. All of that energy that was mobilized in the body to run or fight is frozen there in your physiology and must somehow be discharged. An animal, being unencumbered by logical thought would run away, allow its body to tremble and shake, or otherwise use up this energy until its nervous system returned to normal. In this example you thank the policeman, and then get in his patrol car while he drives you home. The energy you mobilized and then halted with the freezing response is not dissipated and thus remains frozen in your system. Dr. Levine describes the result as follows:

> The difference between the inner racing of the nervous system (engine) and the outer immobility (brake) of the body creates a forceful turbulence inside the body similar to a tornado. This tornado of energy is the focal point out of which form the symptoms of traumatic stress.[5]

Working with Trauma in Rolfing

You can see from the above example that one would not want to enter this "tornado of energy" unaware. Therefore, it is important that any body worker or therapist have a basic understanding of trauma's response in the body and knowledge of how to work with this when it comes up in a session.

I watch for subtle (and sometimes not so subtle) responses in the body that indicate when the autonomic nervous system has been activated. The client may report feeling "weird," maybe slightly nauseous, or a little out of breath. There may be a slight trembling going on in the legs, or the client may feel cold and begin to shiver. Images may come up, for the client, accompanied by emotions. Sometimes, the feeling in the room changes and you know there's been a shift. It is important at this time to stop the physical input of Rolfing and resist the temptation to give verbal input, psychological interpretation, or to try to "fix" things. I find that just calling the client's attention to what she is feeling in her body and then waiting, her body will cycle through to resolution and she will settle naturally, without my having to do anything but be present with her felt experience. At times like this, less is more. The client's body knows what is needed and I have to trust that.

In my intake interview before I begin Rolfing, I specifically ask if my client has ever had any accident, injury or trauma of any kind. It is the rare person who hasn't, although often clients will have totally "forgotten" what I consider to be major traumas until I touch a particular part of the body. In a graphic example of this, I worked with an energetic, highly accomplished and successful woman, who was about forty years old. She had reported no accidents or injuries other than a few minor injuries from playing field hockey during college. Her structure showed a very pronounced, enlarged chest region, as if she was holding her breath. Her legs looked small and immature. After about two sessions of Rolfing she reported to me that she had been kidnapped as a small child and had lived in a series of orphanages for several years before being adopted (the small, immature looking legs). A few sessions later she reported that her sister had been shot before her eyes at

The way to new consciousness is through an eclipse, that is, through the darkening of the consciousness - classically expressed as a depression or introversion shrouded by doubt, feelings of hopelessness, fear, lack of meaning, and a sense that life is being threatened with stagnation and death. Unconsciousness threatens consciousness, but from the conflict that then ensues comes the possibility of a new insight, a higher wisdom, a renewal of life in its fullest sense.

– FRED GUSTAFSON

a drive-in movie (the chest caught on the inhale). She showed no emotion and no autonomic responses, as far as I could tell, while she was reporting this. Meanwhile I was incredulous, thinking to myself, "Holy mackerel! No trauma?!"

At forty years old this woman had developed a compensatory pattern that had mostly worked well for her. She was a perfect example of not dealing with a trauma head-on. I had no desire to break up that pattern unless her body and being were clearly demanding it, and to my knowledge and intuition, she was not demanding it. I could have opened up a real mine field if I had launched full tilt into trying to get major structural change in this woman. We went on for a few more sessions without much change, and eventually I lost touch with her. In this situation my familiarity with the trauma response gave me an important warning signal.

With another client, the insight I was able to apply from Dr. Levine's work was a great help. "Octavian" had been directly struck by lightning in his right side. He was in a coma for several days and said he was "out of the body" but seeing and knowing everything that was happening. When he regained consciousness he had a difficult time reconnecting with himself and the world. Octavian demonstrated a classic case of freezing and dissociation. You can't flee from or fight a direct lightning strike! Immobilization and dissociation was his only defense.

Ever since the accident with lightning, Octavian reported that he had been in another accident each year. When I began to Rolf him I noticed that he was quite spacey and dreamy giving a feeling of barely being present, particularly in the right side of his body. It was as if he had jumped out of his right side and was residing in his left. Working very slowly I continually called his attention to the right side of his body and how it felt compared to the left, using the Rolfing touch to help him to regain a felt sense of his body. Slowly Octavian began to re-inhabit the right side of his body as he became more grounded through his feet and more balanced right to left. By the time we had completed the Ten Sessions he was much more present, aware, alert, and able to feel more confidence in fully inhabiting his body again.

Most Rolfers do not have the expertise to do a full-blown trauma negotiation session, called Somatic Experiencing®, as developed by Dr. Levine. In my experience it's too much of a juggling act to try to do both things, and is a good example of needing to work within the parameters of one's training. However, knowing these few basic skills – recognizing trauma reactivation, stopping further intervention, directing the client to her own felt sense of her body, and trusting the wisdom of her body to come to resolution – a Rolfer can assist his client on the way to healing.

* * *

Rolfing works directly with bringing structure to a higher level of order. As Rolfers we are introducing energy into the fascial system with the pressure of our hands at levels which the client is able to assimilate – a process that is ongoing. With a basic understanding of the trauma mechanism, we are able to hold the space for the client to do the same thing, as he or she tunes into the body and slowly begins to allow the deep thawing of the frozen, immobilized energy of past trauma.

The most beautiful thing we can experience is the mysterious. It is the source of all true art and science.
– ALBERT EINSTEIN

Endnotes, Chapter 11

[1] Levine, Peter A., class notes 1991.
[2] Oertel, Paul and Nancy Spanier. Interview. Boulder, Colorado. March 6, 2004.
[3] Levine, Peter A. with Ann Frederick. *Waking the Tiger: Healing Trauma.* Berkeley, California: North Atlantic Books, 1997, 17.
[4] Ibid., 16, 17.
[5] Ibid., 20.

Part IV
The Research

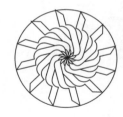

12
Research

As we have seen in previous chapters the interrelationships between body, mind and environment make research on Rolfing difficult and challenging. Both as Rolfers and as clients we feel and see the changes in the being from Rolfing, but how do we capture this intricate dance and look at it under the microscope of science? Different paradigms can be used to approach any research on Rolfing, and Dr. Rolf relates to this when she speaks of her interest in the five levels of thinking offered in Gaston Bachelard's book, *The Philosophy of No*. Dr. Rolf, Emmett Hutchins, and Peter Melchior used Bachelard's epistemological profile in their lectures to illustrate various ways of considering knowledge and science. My class notes from Emmett Hutchins explain these levels as follows:

Level One

Level one is based on direct sensory experience. When I jump into the lake, the water feels cold. When I pick up a rock, my kinesthetic sense tells me that the rock feels heavy. I know something is so because I feel, see, hear, smell, or taste it.

Level Two

This level of thinking involves comparative measurement. I get a thermometer and measure the temperature of the water. It is 70 degrees. The water isn't considered cold by that measurement, yet it feels cold to me. I weigh the rock and it weighs five pounds. That is not very heavy compared to a rock that weighs fifty pounds but when I pick it up, it feels heavy to me.

Level Three

After observing and measuring phenomena, scientists then come up with a law based on cause and effect. The rock weighs five pounds but this is because you are in the gravitational field of the earth. This level of thinking comes from the left hemisphere of the brain and is more analytical. This third level of thinking is the level of Newton's laws and the principles of mechanics that was the science of the times before Einstein's theory of relativity.

Level Four

Level four involves relationship. The rock only weighs five pounds in relationship to where I am – earth or space. The water, even though it measures 70 degrees feels cold in relationship to my body temperature of 98.6 degrees. In Rolfing we look at the relationships throughout the body. Rather than trying to find the cause of a client's sore shoulder, for example, we look at how that shoulder relates to the rest of the body.[1]

Dr. Rolf described Level Four as the level on which Rolfers should live.

Life is not a straight line. Words come out in a straight line, and therefore a great deal of our education is pretty much linear...Life itself is much more complicated; relationship is a key...You have to begin to look at different relationships, and one of the ways you can look at them is that when a muscle or any structure has been overstressed and shortened, it gets a skewed relationship. The whole Gestalt changes. Relationship is the determinant.[2]

And again:

If you've got to live in a stable world, you'd better quit Rolfing. Your stability lies in appropriate relationships, and that is all."[3]

Level Five

In some ways level five looks like level one. I just know, or intuit, or have an insight about something. If I try to describe it, it will sound like level one. However, the experience of knowing that is experienced in level five does not involve the five senses. This fifth level is the domain of mystical experience, synchronicity or intuition. Many intuitive flashes of insight that have become the basis for new ideas about the nature of reality have come from this level. Einstein's theory of relativity is an example of the fifth level of thinking. Tom Wing has surmised that the Ten-Session Series of Rolfing was discovered by Dr. Rolf as an insight, and Peter reports that Dr. Rolf actually told him that this was the case.[4]

* * *

The challenge in doing research on Rolfing is twofold: first, how does one set up an experiment that is going to prove something in the cause and effect realm, yet one that actually takes place in the realm of relationships? Second, how does one report, in the linear realm of words, something that has taken place at another level?

Dr. Rolf dearly wanted her work to be accepted in the scientific world. Beginning in 1969 her wishes were fulfilled. The preliminary study of the Agnews State Project led to a large study by

In a few decades scientists have gone from a conviction that there is no such thing as an energy field around the human body, to an absolute certainty that it exists. Moreover, science is explaining the roles of energy fields in health and disease. The main reason for the recent change in outlook is the development of sensitive instruments that can detect the minute energy fields around the human body.
– JAMES OSCHMAN, PH.D.

Valerie Hunt and Wayne Massey that actually managed to touch on all five levels of thinking mentioned above. Although there are several other studies on the effects of Rolfing, I have chosen to report on these two, as they seemed to me to be the most far reaching of all the research done on Rolfing over the years.

The Agnews State Project – "Stress, Stimulus Intensity Control, and the Structural Integration Technique."[5]

In 1965 Julian Silverman became the director of research at Esalen Institute in Big Sur, California. He had come from the National Institutes of Mental Health and had authored many papers on subjects such as perception, altered states, shamanism and schizophrenia. With Richard Price of Esalen, Silverman conceived of a new approach of treating schizophrenia and he began this work at Agnews State Hospital in California.[6] In 1969 Silverman decided to organize a project to study the effects of Rolfing. Rosemary Feitis describes this project in *Ida Rolf Talks*:

> We knew from experience that the results [of Rolfing] were dramatic, but the unrolfed world "outside" was often skeptical…The 1969 project was ambitious: brain waves, psychological profiles, blood and urine samples were all tested before, during, and after ten hours of Rolfing. In addition Dr. Valerie Hunt of the UCLA Movement Behavior Lab measured muscle potential at different locations in the body during various activities. All the work was donated by the researchers – Val Hunt and her staff came to San Jose, Julian persuaded the state mental hospital there to lend us space and their brain wave lab and personnel, blood and urine tests were carried out and analyzed in another lab, Dr. Rolf and her staff of one

[Peter Melchior] took care of the Rolfing and conquered logistics.[7]

Silverman and other researchers had discovered that people under an unusual amount of stress, such as schizophrenics and depressives, do not modulate sensory stimuli in the same way as ordinary people do. In previous studies, Silverman and others had explored the "...relationships between *stress, responsiveness, emotionality, motor activity*, and the ways in which individuals *modulate sensory* stimulation."[8] "Electrophysiological studies of sensory functioning have indicated that unique patterns of modulating sensory stimulation are associated with differences and degree and kind of psychological stress."[9]

Their hypothesis was that Structural Integration would have some measurable physiological and emotional effect that would show how well the subjects were able to modulate environmental stimulation. In a report on this project, Silverman summarizes the conclusions:

> The research review here suggests that when the musculoskeletal structure is properly balanced, the central nervous (communication) system functions more efficiently. In turn, energy is utilized more economically by the musculoskeletal system and receptivity and sensitivity to the environment are increased. Even in so-called normal individuals, when core physical structures are relatively undifferentiated, there is an identifiable lack of stability in sensory and motor transmission. This, up to now elusive instability at the physical core, serves to maintain a subtle imbalance in neural transmission (and visa versa) and therefore in over-all adaptation.[10]

In a sense, the electro-magnetic pattern creates a mold, which is eventually filled by matter, giving rise to a tangible, material body. Both the material body and the field have their own "brains," but the life-field brain is nothing like the physical brain; it's more of an organizing pattern that maintains the structure of an organism and also instructs the body's new cells– the ones that replace those cells constantly dying within us– where they belong in the human body.

– ROBERT FULFORD, D.O.

Valerie Hunt and Wayne Massey, "A Study of Structural Integration from Neuromuscular, Energy Field, and Emotional Approaches" 1977.[11]

Many times, while Rolfing, I have wondered about what might be going on in the physiology under my hands. *Wouldn't it be wonderful to have x-ray eyes to see into the body!* I have thought. Some answers to my questions were provided in a study by Valerie Hunt and Wayne Massey. Their research involved a wide spectrum of observations – from anxiety levels, muscular performance, and how one processes information, to blood and urine tests. Using a nationally-known aura reader, Roselyn Bruyere, this study investigated an entirely different way of seeing. Although Bruyere would be looking at the energy field around the body, not into the structure like an x-ray, still the information she provided turned out to be remarkable.

The Agnews State Project set up the scientific protocols for this Hunt-Massey study, a more extensive investigation covering five years. Dr. Valerie Hunt, a kinesiologist and author of *Infinite Mind: The Science of Human Vibrations* (1995), was the first to scientifically validate the existence of the human energy field and its vibrational patterns during pain and disease, as well as during emotional and spiritual states. Her experiences with Emilie Conrad Daoud, a dancer and shamanic healer, had led Hunt to become interested in human energy fields. Even though she is essentially a scientist, holding advanced degrees in psychology and physiological science from Columbia University, her own personal experiences contributed to many of her explorations in these areas.[12]

My background in neurophysiology and psychology neither prepared me to understand nor be interested in parapsychological happenings. So my introduction to energy field phenomena had to be serendipitous. I had taught at Columbia University, the University of Iowa, and U.C.L.A. where I researched skilled and pathological muscular activity, the movement behavior of individuals, and the neuromuscular patterns of emotions...To my surprise, data showed related patterns between neuromuscular behavior and personality. The individual's movements shadowed his unique personal characteristics. But other strange information emerged that did not fit with accepted physiology.[13]

Later on, Dr. Hunt noticed at a student dance concert that she attended at U.C.L.A. that many of the dancers moved especially well, almost like professionals. Upon questioning them later, she discovered that these dance students attributed their improved performance to having been Rolfed.

The body is shaped, disciplined, honored, and in time, trusted.

– MARTHA GRAHAM

Now we know that connective tissue has piezoelectric capacities, which can act like an electrical system, where stretching enhances the electrical capacity. Therefore we conjectured that connective tissue was more than tissue scaffolding. It seemed to dictate the flow of electromagnetic energy throughout the body at the finest level.

With curiosity I conducted studies and discovered that after Rolfing, muscles did contract more smoothly and with less effort. People moved more efficiently. (Hunt, 1972) But at that time there was no known objective method to evaluate their subjective feelings of health, vitality and consciousness.[14]

Dr. Hunt continued her exploration of effects of Rolfing by using electromyography, and these preliminary studies established the groundwork and protocol for the 1977 Hunt-Massey project.

Forty-eight subjects were divided into two groups of twenty-four each. Both groups were equally composed of men and women, each of whom met the established experimental criteria for being a subject in the study. One group served as the control. From the other, the experimental group, four subjects were selected for study during the Rolfing sessions. These subjects, two men and two women, were called "experimental group two." The twenty-four subjects in the experimental group were given the complete Ten-Session Series of Rolfing over a five-week period.[15]

Energy is the real substance behind the appearance of matter and forms.

– RANDOLPH STONE, D.O., D.C., N.D.

Both experimental and control subjects were evaluated before and after the five week period by the following procedures: State-Trait Anxiety Inventory (STAI); EEG recordings of right and left hemispheres while resting, sorting blocks and mathematical calculations; EMG recordings of six daily living tasks; energy field photography (Kirlian) and DC field recordings. The four experimental group subjects were further evaluated during Rolfing by: DC field recordings, and electronic recording of the chakra locations simultaneously with an aura reader's [Rosalyn Bruyere] continuous report of the auric field.[16]

The results of this study were truly fascinating, especially considering that this study was done about thirty years ago. I refer you to the write up in the abstract, but briefly the results were as follows:

- a decrease in the anxiety state, more calm feelings of well being

- muscular actions and specific tasks were performed more skillfully
- less fatigue and more conservation of energy
- an increase in right-hemisphere brain dominance when needed for right-brain activity
- changes in thought processes and ways of processing data
- greater movement efficiency
- improved balance and organization of the neuromuscular system resulting in improved efficiency of movement.
- Rolfing was postulated to affect the concept of time and its duration. [17]

As if these findings alone weren't enough, the results of the electronic and auric field study with "experimental group two" seemed to be the most remarkable of all. These were enthusiastically reported by Dr. Hunt in *Infinite Mind*, by Rosemary Feitis in *Ida Rolf Talks*, and by Peter Melchior (who was one of the participating Rolfers with Dr. Rolf) in his interview with me. Briefly:

- the energy flow in the chakras increased
- the auric colors brightened
- the aura reader saw light-blended colors in the aura – such as peach, pink, ice blue, and violet – that had not been reported before
- the fields of the Rolfer and Rolfee interacted with each other during the Rolfing
- the subjects' energy fields responded to emotional states
- the subjects reported memories and images when certain areas of their bodies were Rolfed.[18]

According to Dr. Hunt:

Although the muscular changes from Rolfing were sub-
stantial (Hunt 1972), the energy field data were spectacu-
lar. The findings established clear cut parameters for future
study and provided consistent results that have held up in
ensuing research…The upward energy flow in the chakras
progressively increased during the Ten Sessions. In the
beginning the energy was small, dark in color, low in frequency and amplitude with an uneven flow. During later
sessions the energy was even, light in color, with a higher
amplitude and frequency.[19]

As a result of the Rolf study, we discovered energy
emanations from the body's surface beyond the frequencies
of the neuromuscular system. At the present time the only
appropriate explanation is the existence of a bioenergy
field…Although sensitives throughout history have
described auric emanations, this is the first reported objective, electronic evidence which validates their subjective
observations of auric color discharges…In other words, we
could differentiate between primary and secondary colors
by reading the electronic signal shapes.[20]

From Rosemary Feitis in *Ida Rolf Talks:*

She [Dr. Hunt] again used electrodes measuring muscle
potential at various locations, leaving them in place during the Rolfing process. There were, in addition to this
constant monitoring, trained witnesses to the process – a
Rolfer and an "aura reader." They found that three kinds
of observations tallied – what the Rolfer saw as a topo-
graphical and spatial change, what the aura reader saw as
an energy-color change, and what Val [Hunt] recorded as

a pattern readout on an oscilloscope. Each time the aura reader saw blue, for example, Val's monitors would show a typical pattern; when the Rolfer found that a change had stabilized, both the aura reader and Val's oscilloscope would show a resting color.

It was an exciting project for a number of reasons. For one thing, it showed that Rolfing changes could be monitored on several dimensions, one of which was the "energy body," and that these dimensions were consistent with each other. Furthermore the Rolfing process was used as an opportunity to show that the perceptions of an aura reader were correlated with other measurements of physical change.[21]

From my interview with Peter Melchior:

The Agnews State project was my introduction to serious science. That was the pilot project that led to Valerie Hunt's study. When we started with the project I thought this would be a big "science" thing at U.C.L.A, but the first person I met was Rosalyn Bruyere [an internationally known aura reader] who was going to be my partner on this project. I thought, "This is outrageous! What are these ladies up to?" Nevertheless, the science was impeccable, even with all this other stuff [aura reading and energy fields] going on. I think the most important thing that happened, and Valerie [Hunt] would agree with me because we talked about it not long ago, was that she found that she could predict what Rosalyn [the aura reader] was going to say from looking at the oscilloscopes. There was a precise oscilloscopic wave that was for blue, and there was another one for yellow; one was kind of a spike and one was a sine wave, and green was a combination of the two. One of

Everyone inhabits a reality of non-change lying beyond all change. The experience of this reality brings change under our control.

– DEEPAK CHOPRA M.D., *AGELESS BODY TIMELESS MIND*, 33.

the other things that happened was that colors showed up [in the aura of the subjects] – we have no idea what this means – that were never seen in the human aura before. When we got into sessions eight, nine and ten, [Rosalyn] was beginning to see pastels like peach and cream that she'd never seen in a body before and she had been reading auras all her life. So that was exciting! But none of it was exciting in a way that could actually be used to promote Rolfing.[22]

Dr. Rolf's Work with Children

A three-year pilot project was reported in 1981 by Robert Toporek, a Certified Advanced Rolfer. The published report on this project was called "The Promise of Rolfing Children." (This study was previously mentioned with accompanying photographs in Chapter 10, *Special Considerations*.)

For four weeks in the Spring of 1978, Dr. Rolf and five Rolfers Rolfed nine children and four babies. The children were given the basic Ten-Session Series. The babies were Rolfed but did not receive the full Ten Sessions. This project was reported in an anecdotal and pictorial form. The photographs of the changes in these children are quite dramatic. (*See* Figures 12.1 a and b) The parents and the children were interviewed before and after the Rolfing. Some of the children were photographed one year after having completed the Ten-Session Series, but no further Rolfing, and photographed again after two years, also with no further Rolfing. The photographs show how the movement toward more order in their structures continues along a trajectory of increasing order as they grow, even though they had no further Rolfing after the original Ten Sessions.[23] Toporek reported that some parents found that remarkable changes took place in their children:

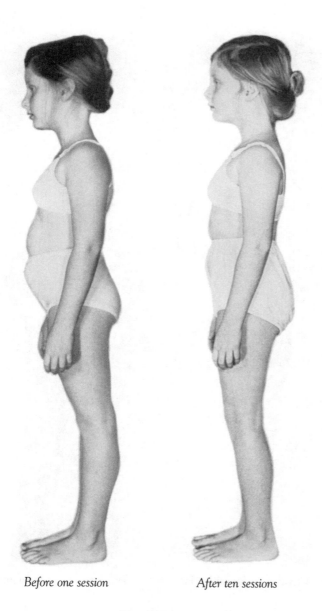

Before one session   *After ten sessions*

Figure 12.1a
"Jo" in four stages
From The Promise of Rolfing Children *by Robert Toporek. Used with permission.*

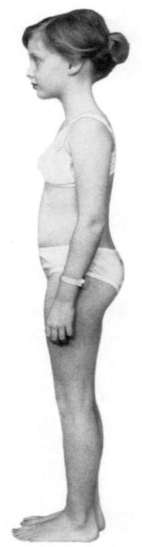 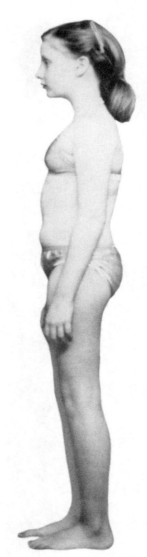

One year later with no further Rolfing   *Two years later with no further Rolfing*

Figure 12.1b

Jo's mother insisted that we mention the effect Rolfing has had on Jo's creativity. She says, "when Jo was born, I knew that this child would be a creative spiritual child." Since her Rolfing Jo has flourished in this regard. Rolfing seems to have given her a centeredness she never had before. This has increased her ability to direct her creative energies. Her creativity, her mother reports, has developed in many areas. She plays the violin, sings, dances, appears in plays, and does art work.[24]

PAUL'S STORY

Paul is a dancer, actor, singer, teacher of expression and Jin Shin Jyutsu practitioner. His story demonstrates that one must work with the changes that happen in Rolfing. For Paul, who had learned specific dance forms, his new freedom and alignment required him to relearn how to dance without those particular tension patterns that he had learned. His perseverance is remarkable as you will see by his story. His main Rolfer was Emmett Hutchins, but I also worked with him off and on over the course of the years when I was in Boulder.

It [Rolfing] was always this sense of being put back on track, that wherever I was physically, psychically, spiritually or emotionally, where I felt I was caught in something, that somehow getting a Rolfing session would reacquaint me with something about myself that I needed to know and that I needed to be involved with to stay true to myself. I was working

Ida [Rolf], I believe, had spoken about where, if you take away the tension patterns in the body, people will intuitively set themselves up in proper relationship – in proper relationship to each other and proper relationship between bones, and between muscles. All that sets up harmonious relationships and kinesthetic relationships that are pleasing. And those things happen naturally in bodies that have been Rolfed.

– PAUL OERTEL, DANCER

with dance forms, working with voice forms, working with people, working with myself, and then I
would get a Rolfing session and say "Oh my God,
look where I wound myself tight!" With each session
there were corresponding emotional, psychic, philosophical and spiritual lessons.

When I asked Paul what was especially intriguing to him
about Rolfing he said,

The visceralness of it and the reality of the contact
with the flesh....It's not something that is only in
the mind but is actually very concrete in the experience of the muscle tissue. So I could actually feel
things about myself and feel my resistances, feel
where I'm blocked, feel where I'm afraid. I like that
contact with the reality of who I am through my
own flesh.

I would take this beautiful sense of balance from
the Rolfing session and then I would challenge it by
trying to do all kinds of things with my body that
were very stressful to my body. I've discovered that
emotionally and physically, you create your art interwoven with and as part of your current defense
mechanisms and your neuroses. Your technical abil-
ities can be woven into your defense mechanisms.
So when you take away those defenses and you
become more open, you also take away a certain
kind of technical ability...What I wanted was a
body that, instead of being armored into socially
conditioned patterns, would be responsive to my
emotional mechanism. Essentially I wanted a body

that was liquid, fluid. And then what ended up happening was that my body was liquid and fluid but my emotional system was not mature enough to handle that freedom. I then had a monster of self-reflection, in that my body was always doing things and being things and turning into things that were really expressions of unresolved parts of myself that were disguised under physical tension, under holding patterns and under social conditioning. When you take those away, then suddenly you are revealed as the body shapes to form into your unconscious material.

The issue with balance was unbelievable. I would find my center of balance in a superficial way and the Rolfer was always driving the movement deeper to the more intrinsics. I would do a particular move because I had certain kinds of patterns. And then suddenly I would become open in a new way and didn't feel good doing the old movement and didn't want to do it anymore. So then I spent hours and hours going over the choreography. I'd have to redo and refigure out how to execute it so that it felt good to me. I realized I had been doing the movements unconsciously. That felt O.K. initially, but then once I woke up I said, "That is not in alignment, that doesn't feel right."…The choreographer would give me things to do that were beautiful expressively but they were very hard to do technically. Then my Rolfer would actually help me figure out how to have enough space in my body to do them without strain. There were also times when I got injured in rehearsals and performances, and I'd go to my Rolfer and he would put things back in

How proud and easy we slide in our skin. Extensible, it stretches to fit our farthest reach, contracts to our least flicker, and all in silky silence.
— RICHARD SELZER, MORTAL LESSONS, 115.

alignment – knees, ankles, head, shoulders and so forth – and show me what I had done to myself.

This process of course was certainly also an interesting experiment for the Rolfer, to work in such a direct way with a person involved in professional performance as his work. It was much like the challenge faced by other Rolfers who have worked with Olympic athletes. How can one organize the body in an optimal way and still have the performer or athlete do a top-level job without too much compromise? For Paul, his life's work is to discover how he can perform as authentically as possible without getting caught in cultural conditioning. In my interview with him I asked him how he resolved this conflict between these cultural dance forms and his own creative expression.

I had a kind of breakdown, and I stopped performing for a number of years. It felt like I just gave out physically and emotionally. There were many reasons, of course, but it looked to me like one of them was just the force of my training, my conditioning. I've been on a journey of challenging my own way of being relative to the culture, the art forms, and the movement forms that were my influences, and finally, little by little, giving up the ones that do not resonate with who I am today. Everyday I'm giving up those kinds of conditionings.

Of course I wondered why anyone would want to continue Rolfing under the circumstances he described of having to give up his old forms and start all over again. Paul's reply was as follows:

Because the Rolfing continues to remind me of who I am in my physical body. In other words this journey with culture and pre-established forms has been a learning journey. It's like going through a whole web where I have learned things. It's ultimately about figuring out "how to be me" and be the kind of performer and expressive artist I want to be. I've been experimenting. The Rolfing continues to bring me home to myself.

* * *

The last paragraph of Valerie Hunt's abstract, "A Study of Structural Integration from Neuromuscular, Energy Field, and Emotional Approaches," serves as a fitting closure to this chapter, as well as to our consideration of integration in the gravity field:

We believe the findings of this study of Rolfing by muscular, energy field and emotional approaches are not happenstances or simply highly related gestaltic factors. While the underlying truths which account for these findings are not known, the brain activity, feeling states, and electrical fields of muscle and aura embody synchronicity. And these truths do posit a new description of body reality lying in the frequency pattern of energy. And as such these patterns constitute surface manifestations of a purposeful man-universe hologram. Yet with our time locked language structure we have no vehicle to describe these findings accurately by hologram. Nonetheless the principal investigator envisions that Rolfing like coherent light uncovers and taps into the perfect body hologram and assists subjects to gain access to a primary body reality. At this level of interpretation Rolfing makes a contribution to human evolution.[25]

The Rolf Institute web page on research lists fourteen research projects that have been done on Rolfing. For those interested see: www.rolf.org/about/research.html

Endnotes, Chapter 12

[1] Rolf class notes.
[2] Feitis, Rosemary. Editor. *Ida Rolf Talks About Rolfing and Physical Reality*. New York, N.Y.: Harper and Row, 1978, 46.
[3] Feitis, 85.
[4] Melchior, Peter, interview, Lyons, Colorado, March 4, 2004; and Tom Wing, Olympia, Washington, March 25, 2004.
[5] Silverman, Julian, et. al. "Stress, Stimulus Intensity Control, and the Structural Integration Technique." *Confina Psychiatra* 16:69-79, 1973. [Reprinted by The Rolf Institute]
[6] Internet www.esalen.org/air/essays/julian-silverman.htm)
[7] Feitis, 21-22.
[8] Silverman, 202.
[9] Ibid., 204.
[10] Silverman, Julian. "Dr. Rolf's Agnews Project." Paper with no date or publisher mentioned. Probably The Rolf Institute, 2.
[11] Hunt, Valerie. "Abstract: A Study of Structural Integration from Neuromuscular, Energy Field, and Emotional Approaches." Boulder, Colorado: The Rolf Institute of Structural Integration, 1977.
[12] Hunt, Valerie. *Infinite Mind: The Science of Human Vibrations*. Malibu, California: Malibu Publishing Company, 1995.
[13] Ibid, 10.
[14] Ibid., 12.
[15] Hunt, "Abstract: A Study of Structural Integration from Neuromuscular, Energy Field, and Emotional Approaches."
[16] Ibid., 1-2.
[17] Ibid., 8-10.
[18] Ibid.

[19] Hunt, *Infinite Mind*, 23.

[20] Ibid., 26-27.

[21] Feitis, 22-23.

[22] Melchior, Peter. Interview. Lyons, Colorado. March 4, 2004.

[23] Toporek, Robert. *A Report on a Pilot Project: The Promise of Rolfing Children*. Philadelphia, Pennsylvania: Robert Toporek, 1981.

[24] Ibid., 11.

[25] Hunt, "Abstract: A Study of Structural Integration from Neuromuscular, Energy Field, and Emotional Approaches." 18.

Part VII
The Metaphysics

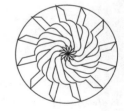

13

The Evolutionary and Transformational Aspects of Rolfing

In the previous chapter on research and Rolfing, we noted that Dr. Valerie Hunt and her research team had essentially discovered a way to measure changes in the human energy field that occurred as a result of Rolfing. According to Emmett Hutchins, it was Dr. Rolf who had asked for the aura reader to be a part of the study, even though this inclusion might have made the study less acceptable to serious scientific researchers. Dr. Rolf, though she might not have mentioned it often, was deeply interested in how the energy body of the human interacted with the gravitational field of the earth, and how that relationship might be enhanced through Rolfing. "The goal of Structural Integration," she said once, "is the creation of order in a three-dimensional body. As this happens we seem to get new insights, new premonitions, greater psychic sensitivity. Structural Integration can change the energy body which is the man."[1]

Emmett touched upon this interest of Dr. Rolf's in an unpublished paper he wrote in 1989:

Mr. Iyengar notes that it is the job of the spine to "keep the brain alert." This means that the spine isn't just a physical structure but a psychological one as well. The moment the front of the spine collapses, the brain collapses, too, and the intense awareness needed for pranayama and meditation vanishes.
— RICHARD ROSEN.
THE YOGA OF BREATH, 102.

If quantum mechanics hasn't profoundly shocked you, you haven't understood it yet.
— NIELS BOHR

During the major portion of her life, Dr. Rolf's overriding personal interest was directed toward yet another field of energy. Here we leave Rolf physics behind and move clearly into metaphysics. We move from her public message into her private teaching which contends that humans are electromagnetic bodies with an electric core and a magnetic sleeve, similar to the earth itself. In an attempt to gain knowledge about this core energy and in pursuit of her interest in personal development, she undertook a study of tantric yoga. As a student of an eastern master, for well over a decade, she carefully examined the teaching for physiological referents. She began to develop an idea. What if, after years of discipline and meditation, one were able to remove all physiological and energetic barriers to the free flow of electric, core energy? And what if one were to place the negative pole of this energized core (root chakra) firmly into the earth while also spanning upward through the positive pole (crown chakra) toward infinity? Would the personal electromagnetic field be reinforced by the field of the earth? Could this not describe a transcendent state of energetic integration between human and cosmos? Could this correspond to awakening of kundalini and the appearance of super-normal powers of mind and body? Are chakras the vortices through which this highly empowered electromagnetic source communicates with matter?[2]

Dr. Rolf's idea of a direct physical intervention with the hands to change structure followed a principle of physics that, when energy is added to a system it affects the order of that system. The tendency for a system to break down and spiral into chaos is called entropy and the tendency of a system to continue to organize itself is syntropy. Adding energy could be in the form of touch and pressure, such as in Rolfing, or it could also be in the form of heat, ultrasound, light, and color.[3] Dr. Valerie Hunt, in her book *The Infinite Mind: The Science of Human Vibrations*, describes a healthy system as one that is open, complex and adaptable. She goes on to describe how the introduction of energy lessens the entropy in the human energy field:

> The new electromagnetic model of illness and health is like this: material tissue ages, gets sick and diseased. It repairs itself, but eventually entropy takes over and causes deterioration and disintegration. This is not true in the human field where, by the introduction of new energy, the field improves, or even becomes more refined. The field is affected before we breathe, eat, or ingest substances, making it the first line of disturbance, defense, and regeneration. Regeneration comes from re-energizing the field, and hence the tissue.[4]

Rolfing re-energizes the field by bringing energy and order to the tissue, which then affects the human energy field. This reflects Dr. Rolf's choice of working on the body on which she could get her hands – the physical body.

The Body as a Laboratory for Transformation

Dr. Rolf mentions, in *Ida Rolf Talks*, that all through the 1920s, when she was in her mid- and late twenties, she studied yoga with an American teacher named Pierre Bernard, who had spent most of his childhood in India and was considered to be a tantric practitioner.[5] Emmett also acknowledges her study of tantric yoga with an Eastern master in the previous quote from his paper.[6] There are various brief indications of her respect for the work of Gurdjieff and her association with J.G. Bennett, who was a primary student of Gurdjieff.

The bioenergy field of health is a palpable sensation to the examining hands of a physician...It is a rhythmic feeling of interchange between the patient's body and his biosphere in which there is a total interchange without any areas of restriction, impaction, trauma, or stress. It is a feeling of total internal and external environmental capacity to express wellness. It is the end point of a physician's treatment program.
– ROLLIN BECKER, D.O.

I find all this particularly fascinating since I have recently met Lee Lozowick, a Western Baul spiritual master, who is deeply knowledgeable in Eastern tantra. The Bauls of Bengal, India, were a sect of singers and dancers who used their art and music as ecstatic devotional worship of the Divine.[7] The connection of this to Dr. Rolf's work, for me, is in the attention paid to the inherent knowledge and wisdom of the body. To quote from *The Hohm Sahaj Mandir Study Manual*, which details the teaching of Lee Lozowick:

> The Bauls are concerned primarily with spiritual practice or endeavor and not with any system of abstract speculation. In this practical aspect, the whole of Baul spiritual practice is based on a belief that the human body is the container of truth....The Bauls believe that God dwells within the human body and is realized only through the body. The Bauls believe that God cannot be found outside the body; in order to realize God, one has to turn to the body itself. This is the essence of one of the basic tenets of Lee's teaching: the body knows.[8]

My class notes from Emmett contain references to Dr. Rolf's idea of a new model of the human being. This new human would no longer have to fight to survive and protect himself or herself. He or she would thus be able to stand tall and free on a narrower base of support, rather than a wide stance ready for attack. The new "man" would not be afraid of his own death and would be free of guilt and shame. This would be reflected in his body, by organization around a vertical line of intention – a lifting up through the top of the head, while remaining grounded through the feet. Dr. Rolf's ideal was that this sense of lift would become natural and easy. As the body begins to lengthen through Rolfing, the energy centers in the body, or chakras, have less static, and the exchange between the material and non-material world that occurs at these centers becomes easier.[9] A body with less static makes subtle levels of awareness more apparent, and thus the inherent knowledge contained within the body more accessible. It would seem to follow that using this kind of a body as a laboratory for discovery would bring forth different results than using a body that was constricted by and locked into past history.

The Mind of the Cells

A 1981 book excited the interest of a lot of Rolfers. *The Mind of the Cells: or Willed Mutation of Our Species* was written by Satprem, a close associate of The Mother (originally named Mirra Alfassa) and Sri Aurobindo. Mother and Aurobindo were working with the evolution of the body, and actually the species of man, through the consciousness of the cells. This seemed in some ways remarkably like Dr. Rolf's vision of a new man. As did Dr. Rolf, Mother felt that the key to a higher order of being and consciousness lay directly in the material (physical) body. With Sri Aurobindo's inspiration and guidance, The Mother embarked on a personal lifetime experiment in physical transformation, which was recorded in detail through her student Satprem, in thirteen volumes, known as *Mother's Agenda* between 1951 and 1973. This was right around the time when Dr. Rolf's work was becoming better known.

"Salvation is physical," said Mother. "Evolution is undoubtedly materialistic, or at any rate material."[10] "The body is the bridge. The body, that is, the cells."[11] "It seems that one can truly understand only when one understands with the body."[12]

At the same time in the 1950s Dr. Rolf was proclaiming: "Rolfing is a road to personal evolution. Metaphysics extends the boundaries of and usually prophecies physics. We are a school of thought. If we can accept that the external world is always

The true aim of life is to find the Divine's Presence deep inside oneself and to surrender to It so that It takes the lead of the life, all the feelings and all the actions of the body.

— THE MOTHER

a projection from the world of thought and ideas, think of our function as Rolfers."[13]

The mind of the cells…what a concept!…that the very cells and atoms of all matter have a consciousness, and that the cells and atoms of our physical body can learn to let go of being programmed by thousands of years of history and habits; never mind letting go of the habits, history, and mechanical functioning of just this one lifetime. Mother seems to be saying that consciousness or life force resides in the cells and atoms of physical matter, and that the mind has dictated how those cells should function. The mind has taught those cells over thousands of years how to be afraid, to believe in illness, harm and death, and to function in a totally mechanical and unspontaneous way. Yet, in their natural way of functioning, cellular consciousness could not even know these imprisoning thoughts, and thus would be free of personal, cultural, or even species history.

Mother goes on to say: "What the body is learning is this: to replace the mental rule of intelligence by the spiritual rule of consciousness. And that makes such a tremendous difference to the point that it increases the body's capabilities a hundredfold. When the body follows certain rules, however broad they may be, it is a slave to those rules, and its possibilities are limited accordingly."[14]

By distinguishing between intelligence and consciousness, and based in her experience, Mother is pointing to a universal consciousness, or as Einstein called it, a Unified Field Theory, present in all matter. The physical mind, however, can place layers or nets on top of this consciousness, obscuring the totally spontaneous functioning that is possible for the cells. The Mother experienced that when one goes deeply *into* the body, instead of escaping out, that it is possible to literally teach the cells how to function from this universal consciousness again.

Dr. Rolf was approaching such a shift in consciousness from the more gross layers of the physical body by reorganizing the fascia.

Since the dawn of history, every civilization has sought to define life's spiritual side. These efforts have led to diverse results, from a pantheon of anthropomorphic gods to the worship of primeval nature or of a single, great deity. To my mind, what is spiritual in the world is the universal source of this cosmic electrical energy, this life force that keeps us all alive.

– ROBERT FULFORD, D.O.

She surmised and showed that by removing outer restrictions in the connective tissue, deeper layers near the center will reorganize, and deeper layers include the cells.

I have always noticed when I am Rolfing that at the simplest bottom-line level, something is not moving – rather, something is stuck. When I reach into the tissue I want to feel resilience, stretchiness, a sense that even the cells are moving. Satprem speaks here that, at the deepest levels, all life is movement.

> It is a fact that all physical theories attempting to explain the structure of our universe and the composition of matter use the wavelike or sinusoidal movement as a sort of constituent and dynamic foundation of physical reality. Whether in electromagnetic or gravitational fields or in atomic interactions, in the heart of the atom or at the ends of our universe, everything moves and propagates as "waves."[15]

Back in the early eighties, when I was deep into Rolfing, I wrote a brief unpublished paper called "Layers and Edges" in which I noted my own experiences of this "all life is movement" phenomenon, both as a Rolfing practitioner and as a receiver of the work:

> All pain, illness, and imbalance in the physical body are due to constriction, contraction, and hanging on to a preconceived form – a form which is too small to contain the experience of the space in front of the spine. Sharp physical edges crowd the cells too densely. This curtails the flow of energy and life force, causing curves, rotations, and other labels of pain and illness. The body should be defined more with gentle planes and arcs rather than edges, as the shadow looks like a line between light and

dark, but on close examination you find there is no demarcation, but a blending. Thus should we relate to our environment. Separateness, our basic fear and basic tool to keep ego intact, causes a pulling in of the body and a sharp demarcation of physical edges that is limiting. Organization of the body in relationship to itself and to vertical demands space. A body that impinges on the space in front of the spine engenders judgment, comparison, competitiveness, and fear. One must allow the rigid outer shell of the body to relax and expand to take up its natural space. This involves relaxing the concepts around which the edges were created. A joyful person is one whose physical shell has expanded enough to allow the natural dancing of the cells. A joyless person has sharp edges and a contracted form that pushes the cells together so closely their dancing is curtailed.[16]

My reflections in "Layers and Edges," as in much of those of The Mother and Dr. Rolf, were attempts at describing an experience and do not necessarily represent anatomical and physiological accuracy. There are certain experiences that lie within a different paradigm than that in which much of science, or even language, operates. Yet, there has to be a place where science and spirituality, the manifest and the unmanifest, meet and integrate. In the following quote Mother states a basic tenet of tantra, which is the non-rejection of anything:

What I have learned: the religions have failed because they were divided, they each wanted you to be religious to the exclusion of other religions; and all knowledge has failed because it was exclusive; and man has failed because he was exclusive. What the new consciousness wants: no more divisions. Being able to understand the extreme spiritual nature, as well as the extreme material nature, and to find their meeting point where…they become a real force.[17]

Is it possible that this "meeting point" of which Mother speaks is the "Line" of Dr. Rolf? Might this be the place where the conscious will of the being to connect to a vertical line through an integrated body can actually become a personal path of evolution?

Rolfing as a Form of Alchemy

We have spoken of Rolfing being a tool, only one of many, for transformation. Transformation involves a change in form and this brings us to the subject of alchemy. The connection between alchemy and Rolfing would lie in the transformation that goes on physically in the body. In addressing the question, does Rolfing have real transformational aspects to it?, let's first look at a distinction between "Transformation" and "transformation" that is given in the *Hohm Sahaj Mandir Study Manual*:

Alchemy is the science of sublimation (making things more sublime), specifically the technology of transforming base substances of lesser value into refined substances of greater value. To understand this further, we must remember that there are two forms of transformation. Transformation with a capital "T" can be envisioned as vertical motion into a new plane, a radical change of context from dualistic to nondualistic. Vertical Transformation is the ultimate intention behind every alchemical gesture. However it continues to prove valuable to use the word "transformation" with a small "t" to indicate change of a nonlinear nature, even though the change may be lateral rather than vertical.[18]

A person's evolvement is based on the development of his or her will. Remember, the mind possesses both desire and will. Everyone must ask, what am I going to put my willpower behind?
– ROBERT C. FULFORD, D.O., *DR. FULFORD'S TOUCH OF LIFE*, 169.

Inherent in alchemy is the fact that the original form must change if you want something new to occur. Even though my brief search on the Internet brought up 109 specific steps in alchemy to change base metal into gold, there are three basic steps mentioned in the *Hohm Sahaj Mandir Study Manual* that are useful when considering the possibility of Rolfing enhancing transformation:

> In general, alchemical processes involve three phases. The initial phase of course, is the set of present conditions. We may depart from the relatively known and stable present conditions and enter into a phase as a result of accepting certain invitations. The middle phase...is where changes take place. Finally the third phase is entered where the new conditions stabilize – keeping in mind that the new conditions may allow for a completely different functionality from the original state. After some degree of stabilization or digestion has occurred, we re-enter the first phase or "ready" position again.[19]

The second phase of "depart[ing] from the relatively known and stable present conditions" often happens, and actually should happen to varying degrees during the Ten-Session Series of Rolfing. Quoting from the *Manual* again: "As rough as it sounds, the purpose and necessity of the in-between state [the second phase] are clear. Change cannot occur without it. Since a system's form determines its functionality, if a function is to change, its form must change...Predispositions must re-order to allow something new to occur."[20] It could almost be Dr. Rolf saying this!

Rolfing involves a certain level of "taking apart" in order to come together in a new way. Old armoring must be released in order to address the aberrations that have formed at deeper layers. The genius of the Rolfing Ten-Session Series is that it specifically takes you through the stages of moving from the hard solid state through a loosening and dissolving of the old form, to a new form and a new order. This dissolution can feel pretty weird sometimes, but there are specific integrating techniques in Rolfing that help a client to deal with this "neither here nor there" feeling as he or she goes through the process of change. One technique could be as simple as changing the pattern in an ankle that has been continually strained and then locked in that abberated position. The Rolfer will first soften the defense system of hard, unoxygenated tissue and then re-order the ankle in a proper way to relate to the leg. The whole system of the body will then respond in a new way to even this simple change.

The alchemical process of transformation is not an instant, one-time thing, but is ongoing in cycles throughout a lifetime, or lifetimes, until the "base metal" of the separative ego-self has transformed into the "gold" of the true Divine Self.

As we have already ranged far out in our explorations in this chapter, let's go a little farther out for the fun of it. When traveling in India, Lee Lozowick and a few of his students met a recognized alchemist, a man who has been studying and practicing intensely in this field for decades. Among other things, this alchemist has produced a powerful alchemical gold elixir, called Tonic Gold®. I had the good fortune to interview Tom Lennon, one of Lee's students, who has met this alchemist on several occasions. What Tom has learned from this association could be likened to some of the descriptions by The Mother in the previous quotes from *The Mind of the Cells*. The Mother was working directly with intention and her bodily experience to change cellular programming. She was using her body as a laboratory of discovery and feedback. According to Tom, the Tonic Gold is an alchemical substance that also works at a deep cellular level to release blockages by essentially infusing the cells with light. In a way, Rolfing also infuses the cells with light by providing space and a central organizing principle of the Rolf Line. Tom elaborated for me:

You are an alchemist; make gold of that.
– WILLIAM SHAKESPEARE, *THE LIFE OF TIMON OF ATHENS*

I consider the fluctuation of the cerebrospinal fluid to be the fundamental principle in the cranial concept. The "sap in the tree" is something that contains the Breath of Life, not the breath of air – something invisible. Dr. Still [A.T. Still, founder of Osteopathy] referred to it as one of the highest known elements in the human body, replenished from time to time. Do you think we will ever know from whence it cometh? Probably not. But it is there. That is all we need to know.

– WILLIAM
SUTHERLAND, D.O.

The world of the alchemist is: your body is your laboratory. Your cellular life is what's feeding back information, reporting back to you about what's working, and the context is that this is all about your work with the Divine. It's not about making gold, it has to do with dissolution and the light of the Divine…An alchemist's work is in the body, just like the Bauls of Bengal.[21]

Regarding what the alchemist called his "golden elixir" Tom explained:

This is alchemical gold [potable gold], which he also calls "organic." It is everywhere in the Universe; so he works with it…in all these alchemical processes so that it can become digestible, accessible. It takes the physical side of alchemy and imbues it into your body. Whether you feel it or not it is at work. This [Tonic Gold®] works where it needs to go at the cellular level…He [the alchemist] says that, on the cellular level…this gold has a vibratory force…it moves through the body in such a way that it penetrates resistance. I can only imagine that the resistance is in the form of an energy blockage.

According to Tom Lennon, when one uses intention when imbibing this Tonic Gold it gives far more focus to the cellular changes:

If what is above is below ["as above so below"] – that's what the alchemist said, that's what the Bauls have said – the Universal principles that are at play in the Divine Universe are no different on the cosmic scale than they are on the cellular level. No different. So, when he talks about imbuing your body with this cosmic gold, he's talking

about imbuing your body with this energy, which is actually the primordial energy of the Universe, which in and of
itself you could label the energy of God...

   If an astral body and a subtle body exist, and I have no
reason to deny that they do, they must move; there has to
be [movement] from the gross form into the cellular into...
the atomic – into whatever creates the energetic vibrational forces that may be these other bodies; that's a continuum. We just can't perceive it. But let's just assume it's
true. So the cellular part is only part of the continuum...It
just may be like the nexus, maybe the turning point, the
bridge, the crossover point, in which the subtle becomes
the energetic manifest in physical form. That's my sense of
it.[22]

Those last few sentences are precise in terms of the place on
the continuum from the manifest to the unmanifest where we
might have an effect on our own awareness. The Mother spoke of
the power of intention in transforming cellular consciousness, and
my Rolfing teachers also spoke of how vital it is to believe in what
can happen in Rolfing, and to engage one's client in his or her
own intention for change. Whether it is approached on the
nuclear, atomic, molecular, cellular, or connective tissue levels –
on whatever level of manifestation, changes in one level will
affect all the other levels. The alchemist described above is working at more subtle levels of atomic, molecular, and cellular structure, which in turn will affect structure on grosser levels. Dr. Rolf
is working directly on the body on which she can get her hands.

   Being the direct hands-on type myself, what I particularly like
about Rolfing is that it begins on the gross level of physical structure. As a Rolfer, I get to put my hands directly on the physical
body, and see and kinesthetically feel immediate change. As the
Rolfee, I get to feel the Rolfer's fingers (and sometimes elbow!)

Certitude is seized by some minds, not because there is any philosophical justification for it, but because such minds have an emotional need for certitude.

— ROBERT ANTON WILSON, *THE NEW INQUISITION*.

Ritual is to the internal sciences what experiment is to the external sciences.

— TIMOTHY LEARY

directly in my flesh, and I can use that immediate present-time sensation to wake up and discover how I am holding. I can then intend the Rolf Line through my body and make connections that I wasn't able to make before. From macrocosm to microcosm and back, from manifest to unmanifest and back, there is a current, a connection, an unbroken set of interrelationships. Working anywhere on this continuum will resonate throughout.

Dr. Rolf's more metaphysical and far-reaching ideas for the possibilities of personal growth and development inherent in Rolfing have been touched upon only briefly. As a person deeply grounded and well-studied in physics and the biological sciences, she only hinted at the broader vision she held. A discussion of Rolfing would be incomplete without considering the full breadth and scope of this vision. Emmett Hutchins, as an early student of Dr. Rolf's, a longtime practitioner of the Rolfing, and one who was perhaps most interested in Dr. Rolf's hypotheses of the possible evolutionary aspects of Rolfing, is well qualified to speak of these ideas. I will end this chapter with a quote from Emmett's paper entitled "Structural Integration: A Path of Personal Growth and Development":

What about discipline of mind and spirit? Surely this path of the masters cannot be reduced to mere biophysics. Here Dr. Rolf would suggest that, in addition to whatever spiritual and religious practice might empower an individual, the practitioner of Structural Integration chooses a path of service to his species. And with this service, whether conscious or not, comes refinement of mind and spirit, the ability to "love" in its highest sense. Additionally, the Recipe is the vehicle through which the practitioner focuses and develops clear intention. The Recipe is the ritual and discipline of this path of service.

Dr. Rolf's teachings and hypotheses covered so many areas of inquiry that no one can explore them all with equal intensity. And she certainly never expected most of her students to accept her work in its fully mystical context. So she presented the challenge of her work in many ways more palatable to the practical mind. However, some degree of personal commitment to the idea of self-organization around a vertical line of intention is basic. When she said "Rolfing is a way of life," she implied more than passive reorganization of the fascial body. In a paper written two years before her death, Dr. Rolf states: "The appropriate integration of the bodies of man in the gravity field is a long term evolutionary project. Not even the first page has been turned yet."[22]

Endnotes, Chapter 13

[1] Rolf class notes with Emmett Hutchins.
[2] Hutchins, Emmett. *Structural Integration: A Path of Personal Growth and Development*. Unpublished paper written in 1989, 2-3. Used with permission.
[3] Hutchins, Emmett. Rolf class notes.
[4] Hunt, Valerie. *The Infinite Mind: The Science of Human Vibrations*. Malibu, California: Malibu Publishing Co., 1995, 245.
[5] Feitis, Rosemary. Editor. *Ida Rolf Talks About Rolfing and Physical Reality*. New York, New York: Harper and Row, 1978, 7.
[6] Hutchins, Emmett. *Structural Integration: A Path of Personal Growth and Development*. Unpublished paper, 1989, 3.
[7] *Hohm Sahaj Mandir Study Manual: A Handbook for Practitioners of Every Spiritual and/or Transformational Path Volume II*. Prescott, Arizona: Hohm Press, 1996, 294.
[8] Ibid., 304.
[9] Hutchins, Rolf class notes.
[10] Satprem. *The Mind of the Cells: or Willed Mutation of Our Species*. New York, N.Y.: Institute for Evolutionary Research, 1981, 5.

[11] Ibid., 9.
[12] Ibid., 10.
[13] Rolf, Ida P., class notes from Emmett Hutchins.
[14] Satprem, 152.
[15] Ibid., 23.
[16] Sise, Betsy. *Layers and Edges*. Unpublished Paper, undated.
[17] Satprem, 179.
[18] *Hohm Sahaj Mandir Study Manual: A Handbook for Practitioners of Every Spiritual and/or Transformational Path Volume IV*. Prescott, Arizona: Hohm Press, 2002, 209.
[19] Ibid., 210.
[20] Ibid., 211.
[21] Interview with Tom Lennon. Boulder, Colorado. March 3. 2004.
[22] Hutchins, Emmett. *Structural Integration*, 4.

In Memoriam

June 4th 2005
Peter Melchior's Memorial at
Planet Bluegrass in Lyons, Colorado

We came from all corners – Israel, Brazil, Europe, and all
across the United States to honor him and celebrate the gift of his
life – my dear teacher and friend Peter Melchior. Approximately
three hundred were to gather outside near a river by some cliffs in
a grove of trees, a place Peter had always loved. A large tent was
set up for food. It had poured rain all day until about 3:00 P.M.
when slowly the clouds lifted and the sun flitted intermittently in
and out. As we came back like homing pigeons to the source of
Peter we greeted each other again after years. Tom was there from
Washington and Jan from Santa Fe as well as other teachers and
students from both GSI and the Rolf Institute. Heads were a bit
grayer and children we knew had grown to adults with children of
their own. Forest Melchior greeted me, now a grown woman and
Rolfer in her own right, reminding me that I had given her her
first Ten Sessions when she was fifteen years old. It seemed that
life and death were intertwined in their endless embrace.

We sat together under the trees with the river before us and a
sheer cliff behind the river looming as a backdrop for circling
birds. Nature was the only sound to accompany the voices of

Peter's family as each rose to speak of the tremendous gift of both his life and the last days of his dying process. He was *teacher* till the end, joking and accepting his way on the journey of death with peace and love. His last words were, "I'm alright."

As Forest, Peter's daughter, rose to speak I saw a lovely young woman with tremendous presence and charisma, and thought to myself that she was well on her way to becoming the powerful teacher her father was. I saw a long golden thread – beginning with the work of Ida Rolf herself, threading through the people she had touched, through my teachers to me, and through me to my clients. And this threading process was duplicated hundreds of times over, rolling ever onward in the wave of this work called Rolfing.

The service was closed with all of us standing and holding hands in a great circle the way we used to at the beginning and end of every Rolfing class. And as in our classes, every ending allowed a new beginning.

* * *

SMOKE SIGNALS
by Peter Melchior

An old lion with no teeth
sits quietly at the mouth of his cave.
His memories are neither good nor bad, merely images.

The mind is not as soft as the body
and old songs are more than nostalgia
to the heart still open and beating like a spirit drum.

Our time is not simply over, you know.
It is burned into Mother Earth, leaving a trail for you to follow,
and all her creatures are waiting to follow you.

All your ancestors look into your time
demanding your eventual growth into maturity.
We can leave as legacy only everything we could not do.

The only acceptable payment for the gift of Life
is to live it fully – to say yes, and to mean it.
We leave you here with simple blessings and an awesome
duty.

> – Written on June 4, 1995,
> exactly ten years prior to his Memorial.

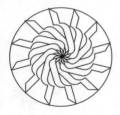

Bibliography

Castaneda, Carlos. *The Eagle's Gift*. New York: Simon and Schuster, Inc., 1981.

_____ *A Separate Reality: Further Conversations with Don Juan*. New York: Simon and Schuster, 1971.

Chopra, Deepak M.D. *Ageless Body Timeless Mind: The Quantum Alternative to Growing Old*. New York: Harmony Books a division of Crown Publishers, 1993.

Clemente, Carmine D. Ph.D. *Anatomy: A Regional Atlas of the Human Body*. Philadelphia: Lea and Febiger, 1975.

Connolly, Lisa. "Ida Rolf." *Human Behavior*. May, 1977.

Cottingham, John T., Stephen W. Porges and Kent Richmond. "Shifts in Pelvic Inclination Angle and Parasympathetic Tone Produced by Rolfing Soft Tissue Manipulation." *Journal of American Physical Therapy Association* vol. 68, no. 9, September 1988.

Cottingham, John T., Stephen W. Porges and Todd Lyon. "Effects of Soft Tissue Mobilization (Rolfing Pelvic Lift) On Parasympathetic Tone in Two Age Groups." *Journal of American Physical Therapy Association* vol. 68, no. 3, March 1988.

Feitis, Rosemary. Interview. New York, March 26, 2004.

_____ Ed. *Ida Rolf Talks About Rolfing and Physical Reality*. New York: Harper and Row, 1978.

_____ Rosemary and Louis Schultz Ph.D. editors. *Remembering Ida Rolf*. Berkeley, California: North Atlantic Books and Boulder, Colorado: The Rolf Institute, 1996.

Feldenkrais, Moshe. *Body and Mature Behavior: A Study of Anxiety, Sex, Gravitation and Learning.* New York: International Universities Press, 1950.

Fulford, Robert C. D.O., with Gene Stone. *Dr. Fulford's Touch of Life: The Healing Power of Natural Life Force.* New York: Pocket Books, a Division of Simon and Schuster Inc., 1996.

Ganong, William F. MD. *Review of Medical Physiology 7ᵗʰ Edition.* Los Altos, California: Lange Medical Publications, 1975.

Guild for Structural Integration: General Information and Training Programs 2001-2005. Boulder, Colorado: Guild for Structural Integration.

Hamilton, W.J. editor. *"The Textbook of Human Anatomy 2ⁿᵈ Edition.* Saint Louis, Missouri: The CV Mosby Company, 1976.

Hammann, Kalen Ph.D. "What Structural Integration (Rolfing) is and Why it Works." *The Osteopathic Physician,* March 1972. Reprinted by the Rolf Institute.

Hay, Louise L. *You Can Heal Your Life.* Santa Monica, California: Hay House, 1984.

Ho, Mae-Wan. *The Rainbow and the Worm: The Physics of Organisms 2ⁿᵈ edition.* Singapore, New Jersey, London, Hong Kong: World Scientific Publishing Company, 1998.

Hohm Sahaj Mandir Study Manual Volume II: A Handbook for Practitioners of Every Spiritual and/or Transformational Path. Prescott, Arizona: Hohm Press, 1996.

Hohm Sahaj Mandir Study Manual Volume IV: A Handbook for Practitioners of Every Spiritual and/or Transformational Path. Prescott, Arizona: Hohm Press, 2002.

Horvitz, Gary. "Ida Rolf, A Retrospective." *Bulletin of Structural Integration* vol. 6, no. 4. Boulder, Colorado: The Rolf Institute, August, 1979.

Hunt, Valerie V. *Infinite Mind: The Science of Human Vibrations.* Malibu, California: Malibu Publishing Co., 1995.

____ and Robert S. Weinberg. "Effects of Structural Integration on State-Trait Anxiety." *Journal of Clinical Psychology* vol. 35, no.2, April, 1979. [Reprinted by the Rolf Institute]

____ "Abstract: A Study of Structural Integration from Neuromuscular, Energy Field, and Emotional Approaches." Boulder, Colorado: The Rolf institute of Structural Integration, 1977.

Hutchins, Emmett. Interview. Kauai, Hawaii, June 9, 2004.

Hutchins, Emmett. "Structural Integration: A Path of Personal Growth and Development." Unpublished paper written for The Guild for Structural Integration in 1989. Used with permission.

Johnson, Don. *The Protean Body: A Rolfer's View of Human Flexibility*. New York: Harper and Row, 1977.

Kirkby, Ron Ph.D. "The Probable Reality Behind Structural Integration: How Gravity Supports The Body." Paper written for a Rolfing class. Boulder, Colorado: The Rolf Institute. Undated.

Korzybski, Alfred. *Science and Sanity: An Introduction to Non-Aristotelian Systems and General Semantics 4ᵗʰ edition*. Lakeville, Connecticut: The International Non-Aristotelian Library Publishing Company, 1958.

Lennon, Tom. Interview. Boulder, Colorado, March 3, 2004.

Lensman, Lana. "Getting it Straight: Scoliosis and Structural Integration." *Massage and Bodywork*, October/November 2003.

Levine, Peter A. with Ann Frederick. *Waking the Tiger: Healing Trauma*. Berkeley, California: North Atlantic Books, 1997.

_____ "Accumulated Stress Reserve Capacity and Disease: An Abstract of a Ph.D. Dissertation."*Bulletin of Structural Integration*. Vol.6, no.2, 14-24. Autumn, 1977.

_____ Class notes from a class on Somatic Experiencing® Boulder, Colorado, 1991.

Linn, Jeff. Interview. Boulder, Colorado. March 5, 2004.

Melchior, Peter. Interview. Lyons, Colorado. March 4, 2004.

Myers, Tom. "Variation in Ida Rolf's 'Recipe'." *The 2004 Yearbook of Structural Integration*. Missoula, Montana: The International Association of Structural Integrators, 2004.

Myss, Caroline, Ph.D. *Anatomy of the Spirit: The Seven Stages of Power and Healing*. New York: Harmony Books, a division of Crown Publishers Inc., 1996.

Oertel, Paul and Nancy Spanier. Interview. Boulder, Colorado. March 6, 2004.

Oschman, James L. Ph.D. "What is Healing Energy? The Scientific Basis of Energy Medicine." A series of articles published in the *Journal of Bodywork and Movement Therapies*. Ed. By Leon Chaitow, ND, DO. New York: Churchill Livingstone, 1996-1998.

Pearce, Joseph Chilton. *The Biology of Transcendence: A Blueprint of the Human Spirit*. Rochester, Vermont: Park Street Press, 2002.

Pert, Candace B. *The Molecules of Emotion: Why You Feel the Way You Feel*. New York: Scribner, 1997.

Robbie, David L. MD. "Tensional Forces in the Human Body." *Orthopedic Review* vol.VI, no. 11, November 1977. [Reprinted by the Rolf Institute]

Rolf class notes from Auditor and Practitioner Rolf Training, Boulder, Colorado, 1977- 1978.

Rolf, Ida P. Ph.D. "An Introduction to Structural Integration." Video film by Robert Pritchard of a lecture given by Dr. Rolf in 1974. The Rolf Institute of Structural Integration.

_____ "The Boy Logan Series." Archival video footage. Rolf Institute, 1977.

_____ *Rolfing: The Integration of Human Structures*. Santa Monica, California: Dennis-Landmine, 1977.

_____ "Rolfing: The Vertical Experiential Side To Human Potential." Blackwood, New Jersey: Ida P. Rolf, 1977.

_____ "Structure: A New Factor in Understanding the Human Condition." A paper presented at The Explorers of Humankind Conference June 10, 1978. [Reprinted by the Rolf Institute]

_____ "Structural Integration: A Contribution to the Understanding of Stress." Reprinted by the Rolf Institute from *Confina Psychiatra* 16:69-79, 1973.

_____ "Rolfing Structural Integration: Gravity: An Unexplored Factor in the More Human Use Of Human Beings." *The Journal of the Institute for the Comparative Study of History, Philosophy and the Sciences*. Vol. I, Number 1, June Issue, 1963.

_____ "What is Rolfing About?" *Bulletin of Structural Integration* vol.6, no.2, 1-3, Autumn, 1977.

Rolf Institute Educational Catalog 2003-2004. Boulder, Colorado: Rolf Institute of Structural Integration, 2003.

Rosen, Richard. *The Yoga of Breath: A Step-by-Step Guide to Pranayama*. Boston: Shambhala, 2002.

Satprem. *Mind of the Cells: or Willed Mutation of Our Species*. New York: Institute for Evolutionary Research, 1981.

Schleip, Robert. "Talking to Fascia – Changing the Brain: A Collection of Articles on Rolfing and the Neuro-myofascial Net." Reprinted from *Rolf Lines* October 1993, pg.1-ll, March 1993, 13-23 and April/May 1991, 25-28. Boulder, Colorado: The Rolf Institute, 1994.

_____ "Fascial Plasticity-A New Neurobiological Explanation Parts I and II." *The 2004 Yearbook of Structural Integration*. Missoula, Montana: The International Association of Structural Integrators, 2004.

Schultz, R. Louis Ph.D. and Rosemary Feitis, DO. *The Endless Web: Fascial Anatomy and Physical Reality*. Berkeley, California: North Atlantic Books, 1996.

Sell, Christina. *Yoga From the Inside Out: Making Peace With Your Body Through Yoga*. Prescott, Arizona: Hohm Press, 2003.

Selzer, Richard. *Mortal Lessons: Notes on the Art of Surgery*. New York: Simon and Schuster, Inc., 1974, 1975 and 1976.

Sheldrake, Rupert. *The New Science of Life: The Hypothesis of Formative Causation*. Los Angeles California: JP Tarcher Inc., distributed by Houghton Mifflin Company, 1981.

Silverman, Julian et. al. "Stress, Stimulus Intensity Control and the Structural Integration Technique."*Confina Psychiatra* 16: 69-79, 1973. [Reprinted by the Rolf Institute]

Silverman, Julian. "Dr. Rolf's Agnews Project." (No date or publisher mentioned. Probably the Rolf Institute)

Smith, Fritz Frederick MD. *Inner Bridges: A Guide to Energy Movement and Body Structure*. Atlanta Georgia: Humanics New Age, 1986.

Sultan, Jan Henry. Interview. Espanola, New Mexico. March 14, 2004.

Toporek, Robert. *A Report on a Pilot Project: The Promise of Rolfing Children*. Philadelphia: Robert Toporek, 1981.

Watson, Craig MD, and Ph.D. *Basic Human Neuroanatomy: An Introductory Atlas 2ⁿᵈ. Edition*. Boston: Little, Brown and Company, 1977.

Wing, Tom. Interview. Olympia, Washington. March 25, 2004.

Photo and Illustration Credits

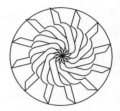

The author gratefully acknowledges the following persons and organizations for granting permission for inclusion of their work in this book.

Frontispiece – Dr. Ida P. Rolf (1897 – 1979), "The Dreamer." Photo by Ron Thompson, used with permission. Contact information: IRolf@aol.com

Dedication page – Peter Melchior (1931 – 2005), photo by Emmett Hutchins, used with permission.

Figure 2.1 – Used with permission of the Rolf Institute of Structural Integration. Contact: www.rolf.org

Figure 2.2 – Drawing by Diana Salles from Schultz, R. Louis, Ph.D. and Rosemary Feitis, D.O. *The Endless Web: Fascial Anatomy and Physical Reality*. Berkeley, California: North AtlanticBooks, 1996, 29. Used with permission.

Figure 2.3 – Photo by Kelly Sell, Prescott Yoga Center, Prescott, Arizona. Contact: www.prescottyoga.com

Figure 2.4 – Photo by Kelly Sell, Prescott Yoga Center, Prescott, Arizona. www.prescottyoga.com

Figure 2.6 – Photos of "J.C." from "A Report on a Pilot Project: *The Promise of Rolfing Children,*" copyright 1981 by Robert Toporek, pages 12 and 13. (No specific credits are given for the photos.) Used with permission of Robert Toporek.

Figure 3.1 – Drawing by Diana Salles from Schultz, R. Louis, Ph.D. and Rosemary Feitis, DO. *The Endless Web: Fascial Anatomy and Physical Reality.* Berkeley, California: North AtlanticBooks, 1996, 26. Used with permission.

Figure 4.1 – Photo by Kelly Sell, Prescott Yoga Center, Prescott, Arizona. www.prescottyoga.com

Figure 4.2 – Photo by Kelly Sell, Prescott Yoga Center, Prescott, Arizona. www.prescottyoga.com

Figures 5.1, 5.2, 5.3 – Photos by Kelly Sell, Prescott Yoga Center, Prescott, Arizona. www.prescottyoga.com

Figures 5.4a and b. – Drawings by John Lodge from Rolf, Ida P. *Rolfing: The Integration of Human Structures.* Santa Monica, California: Dennis-Landman, 1977, 51, 43. Used with permission of Alan Demmerle.

Figure 5.5 – Photo by Kelly Sell, Prescott Yoga Center, Prescott, Arizona. www.prescottyoga.com

Figure 5.6 – This reproduction of "The Outermost Order of Muscles, Side View" is taken from *Albinus on Anatomy* by Robert Beverly Hale and Terence Coyle. New York: Watson – Guptill Publications, 1997, 39. Used with permission.

Figure 5.7 – Drawing by John Lodge from Rolf, Ida P. *Rolfing: The Integration of Human Structures.* Santa Monica, California: Dennis-Landman, 1977, 100. Used with permission of Alan Demmerle.

Figure 5.8 – Drawing by John Lodge from Rolf, Ida P. *Rolfing: The Integration of Human Structures.* Santa Monica, California: Dennis-Landman, 1977, 110. Used with permission of Alan Demmerle.

Figure 5.9 – Drawing by Diana Salles from Schultz, R. Louis, Ph.D. and Rosemary Feitis, D.O. *The Endless Web: Fascial Anatomy and Physical Reality.* Berkeley, California: North AtlanticBooks, 1996, 43. Used with permission.

Figure 5.10 – Drawing by John Lodge from Rolf, Ida P. *Rolfing: The Integration of Human Structures*. Santa Monica, California: Dennis-Landman, 1977, 166. Used with permission. Figure 5.11 – Photo by Kelly Sell, Prescott Yoga Center, Prescott, Arizona. www.prescottyoga.com

Figure 5.12 – This reproduction of "The Fourth Order of Muscles, Front View" is taken from *Albinus on Anatomy* by Robert Beverly Hale and Terence Coyle, New York: Watson – Guptill Publications, 1997, 49. Used with permission.

Figure 7.1 – Ida P. Rolf, "Rolfing Baby." Photo by Ron Thompson, used with permission. Contact information: IRolf@aol.com

Figure 9.1 – Used with permission of the Rolf Institute of Structural Integration. Contact: www.rolf.org

Figures 9.2 a, b, c – Artist and source unknown, tracing by Elyse April.

Figure 9.3 – Keleman, Stanley. *Emotional Anatomy: The Structure of Experience*. Berkeley, California: Center Press, 1985, 147. Used with permission.

Figure 9.4 – Keleman, Stanley. *Emotional Anatomy: The Structure of Experience*. Berkeley, California: Center Press, 1985, 147. Used with permission.

Figure 9.5 a, b – Drawings by Emmett Hutchins, used with permission.

Figure 9.6 – Photo by Kelly Sell, Prescott Yoga Center, Prescott, Arizona. www.prescottyoga.com

Figure 10.1 – Ida P. Rolf, "Eye to Eye." Photo by Ron Thompson, used with permission. Contact information: IRolf@aol.com

Figure 10.2 – "Chris," before and after, from "A Report on a Pilot Project: *The Promise of Rolfing Children*" copyright 1981 by Robert Toporek, page 21. (No specific credits are given for the photos.) Used by permission of Robert Toporek.

Figure 12.1 – "Jo," before and after, from "A Report on a Pilot Project: *The Promise of Rolfing Children*" copyright 1981 by Robert Toporek, pages 10 and 11. (No specific credits are given for the photos.) Used by permission of Robert Toporek.

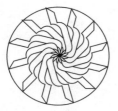

Index

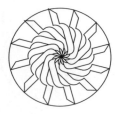

About the Author

Betsy Sise is a graduate of Skidmore College, the University of North Carolina and the University of Arizona. Certified by the Rolf Institute in 1978, she is an Advanced Rolfer with clients in Arizona. Betsy was trained by four of Ida Rolf's earliest students, and from them received a direct communication of the founder's work. She has also studied both dance and yoga, extensively.

Betsy was chairperson of the Admissions Committee, Rolf Institute, and a member of the Education Executive Committee and Board of Directors of the Rolf Institute. A practitioner of meditation, she brings a deep spiritual perspective to her body-work. She lives in Prescott, Arizona.

Information

For information about Rolfing/Structural Integration and Rolf/SI
   Training:
The Rolf Institute website is: http:\ \www.Rolf.org
The Guild for Structural Integration website is:
   http:\ \www.Rolfguild.org

To contact the author, write to: Betsy Sise, c/o Hohm Press, PO Box 31, Prescott, Arizona, 86302, USA

To view the complete Hohm Press Catalog, visit our website at www.hohmpress.com